Special Tests for
Orthopedic Examination

FOURTH EDITION

T0198143

Special Tests for Orthopedic Examination

FOURTH EDITION

Jeff G. Konin, PhD, ATC, PT, FACSM, FNATA
Professor and Chair, Physical Therapy Department
University of Rhode Island
Kingston, Rhode Island
Adjunct Professor, Department of Family Medicine
Primary Care Sports Medicine Fellowship
Brown University
Providence, Rhode Island

Denise Lebsack, PhD, ATC
Associate Professor, Athletic Training
School of Exercise & Nutritional Sciences
San Diego State University
San Diego, California

Alison R. Snyder Valier, PhD, ATC, FNATA
Professor, Athletic Training Programs
Department of Interdisciplinary Health Sciences
Assistant Director, Research Support
Research Professor, School of Osteopathic Medicine in Arizona
A. T. Still University
Mesa, Arizona

Jerome A. "Jai" Isear, Jr., MS, PT, LAT, ATC
Co-Owner, Shoreline Physical Therapy
Wilmington, North Carolina

Holly Brader Marakovits, MPH, RN, BSN, ATC
Coauthor of Second and Third Editions

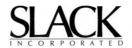

SLACK
INCORPORATED

www.slackbooks.com

ISBN: 978-1-61711-982-8

The procedures and practices described in this publication should be implemented in a manner consistent with the professional standards set for the circumstances that apply in each specific situation. Every effort has been made to confirm the accuracy of the information presented and to correctly relate generally accepted practices. The authors, editors, and publisher cannot accept responsibility for errors or exclusions or for the outcome of the material presented herein. There is no expressed or implied warranty of this book or information imparted by it. Care has been taken to ensure that drug selection and dosages are in accordance with currently accepted/recommended practice. Off-label uses of drugs may be discussed. Due to continuing research, changes in government policy and regulations, and various effects of drug reactions and interactions, it is recommended that the reader carefully review all materials and literature provided for each drug, especially those that are new or not frequently used. Some drugs or devices in this publication have clearance for use in a restricted research setting by the Food and Drug and Administration or FDA. Each professional should determine the FDA status of any drug or device prior to use in their practice.

Any review or mention of specific companies or products is not intended as an endorsement by the author or publisher.

SLACK Incorporated uses a review process to evaluate submitted material. Prior to publication, educators or clinicians provide important feedback on the content that we publish. We welcome feedback on this work.

Published by: SLACK Incorporated
                 6900 Grove Road
                 Thorofare, NJ 08086 USA
                 Telephone: 856-848-1000
                 Fax: 856-848-6091
                 www.slackbooks.com

Contact SLACK Incorporated for more information about other books in this field or about the availability of our books from distributors outside the United States.

Library of Congress Cataloging-in-Publication Data

Names: Konin, Jeff G., author. | Lebsack, Denise, author. | Valier, Alison
   Snyder, author. | Isear, Jerome A., Jr., 1967- , author.
Title: Special tests for orthopedic examination / Jeff G. Konin, Denise
   Lebsack, Alison Snyder Valier, Jerome A. "Jai" Isear, Jr.
Description: Fourth edition. | Thorofare, NJ : SLACK Incorporated, [2016] |
   Preceded by Special tests for orthopedic examination / Jeff G. Konin ...
   [et al.]. 3rd ed. 2006. | Includes bibliographical references and index.
Identifiers: LCCN 2015038145 | ISBN 9781617119828 (paperback : alk. paper)
Subjects: | MESH: Musculoskeletal Diseases--diagnosis--Handbooks. | Physical
   Examination--methods--Handbooks. | Range of Motion, Articular--Handbooks.
Classification: LCC RD734.5.P58 | NLM WE 39 | DDC 616.7/0754--dc23 LC record available at http://lccn.loc.gov/2015038145

Printed in the United States of America.

Last digit is print number: 10 9 8 7 6 5 4

DEDICATION

To John Bond,
may your next phase of life bring you
much happiness and success.
—*Jeff G. Konin, PhD, ATC, PT, FACSM, FNATA*

To my students,
who remind me why I love teaching.
—*Denise Lebsack, PhD, ATC*

To my family, friends, and colleagues.
You all bring much happiness to my life.
—*Alison R. Snyder Valier, PhD, ATC, FNATA*

To Mitzie, Brooks, Harrison, and Jackson,
for being such true blessings in my life.
—*Jerome A. "Jai" Isear, Jr., MS, PT, LAT, ATC*

CONTENTS

ACKNOWLEDGMENTS

When the concept of this handy guide to special tests was conceptualized at Seacrets in Ocean City, Maryland, in 1995, none of us ever dreamed we would be writing a fourth edition some 20 years later.

We continue to extend our gratitude to each of you who have remained supportive of the project. Without your continued valuable feedback, we would not be able to successfully launch an improved version. The world of health care is changing in so many ways, and listening to your many ideas contributes to the valuable improvements that we try to make with each updated edition. It is truly wonderful to talk to so many of you who get excited about the way this handbook helped you get through classroom labs and tests, clinical internships, and ultimately your certification exam. The stories that many of you have shared about this book being the most used and most helpful throughout your career is very humbling.

Twenty years working with the same publisher is also quite an accomplishment. Kudos to the people at SLACK Incorporated. We remain indebted to John Bond (Chief Content Editor) and Peter Slack (President) for believing in our ideas and trusting our foresight. To this day, their support and friendship are second to none. Our sincere thanks go to Jennifer Cahill (Senior Project Editor) and April Billick (Managing Editor) for all of their hard work on this project. Most of all, to Brien Cummings (Senior Acquisitions Editor) for jumping on board like a champion and ensuring that we all stayed on task—not an easy thing to do with a transition of authors residing in different geographical time zones. Despite technology and its added benefits, long distance collaboration still poses challenges.

Special thanks go to the contributors who performed the significant legwork in researching the most current peer-reviewed manuscripts for the special tests included in this edition: Kelsey Picha, MS, ATC, and Steph Trigsted, MS, ATC. Under the guidance of Alison Valier, who spearheaded this fourth edition, Kelsey and Steph performed tedious, yet valuable, work contributing to a significant revision in the format of this edition. This time-consuming and detailed process plays a vital role in the recognition of evidence-based practice. In addition, we would like to thank Casey Hill, DPT, and Justin Jacapraro, ATC, CPT, SPT, for their assistance in reviewing the text, figures, and videos. Finally, we would like to thank Shannon Matheny and Douglas Pizac for graciously posing as examiner and subject for images and videos.

—*Jeff G. Konin, PhD, ATC, PT, FACSM, FNATA*
—*Denise Lebsack, PhD, ATC*
—*Alison R. Snyder Valier, PhD, ATC, FNATA*
—*Jerome A. "Jai" Isear, Jr., MS, PT, LAT, ATC*

About the Authors

Jeff G. Konin, PhD, ATC, PT, FACSM, FNATA is a Professor and the Chair of the Physical Therapy Department at the University of Rhode Island in Kingston, Rhode Island. One of the original authors of this textbook, Dr. Konin is recognized as a Fellow by both the American College of Sports Medicine and the National Athletic Trainers' Association for his contributions.

Dr. Konin has previously held the positions of Director of Athletics at Eastern Connecticut State University, Faculty and Vice Chair of Orthopaedics and Sports Medicine at the University of South Florida (USF), Executive Director of the Sports Medicine and Athletic Related Trauma (SMART) Institute at USF, Director of the Graduate Athletic Training Program at USF, and Health Sciences Faculty and Assistant Athletic Director for Sports Medicine at James Madison University. Dr. Konin is also founding partner in The Rehberg Konin Group, a firm providing consulting in the areas of sport safety and education, and a founding member of Sport Safety International, specializing in the delivery of sport safety educational resources.

Dr. Konin's published work and invited presentations have focused in the area of sports medicine with a particular interest in injury prevention and sport safety. He has shared his expertise at professional conferences throughout the United States, as well as in Australia, New Zealand, Italy, Norway, Romania, England, and Austria. His experiences have included serving on the medical staff for the 1996 Olympic Games and as a medical coordinator for the USA Wheelchair Rugby Paralympic Team.

Denise Lebsack, PhD, ATC has been an Associate Professor of Athletic Training in the School of Exercise & Nutritional Sciences at San Diego State University (SDSU) since 1994. During much of that time she has served as the Athletic Training Program Director, and has coordinated 3 separate Self Study Reports for the Athletic Training Education Program's accreditation. As part of that process and her role as an athletic training educator, Dr. Lebsack has developed a philosophy that seeks to optimize student learning and educational outcomes. Her goal is to provide students with educational tools that aid in the learning process and that instill academic inquiry and understanding. When Dr. Konin first approached her with the original book idea, she immediately knew it was a project that fit perfectly with her educational philosophy and goals for her students.

In keeping with these goals, Dr. Lebsack was also an author for a 2-disc CD-ROM series on special tests used during the injury evaluation process that incorporated video demonstration and anatomical representation of a positive test result. Her interest in instructional technology led to several published articles evaluating the effectiveness of technology in the classroom. Given her research and experience as an educator, she was invited to be a Guest Editor for the *Journal of Athletic Training*'s Special Issue on "Athletic Training Education" (2002;37[4]). She has also coauthored the textbook *The Athletic Trainer's Guide to Strength and Endurance Training*.

Dr. Lebsack currently spends her time focused on the classroom and engaging students in the learning process. She serves as a faculty advisor for the SDSU student organization Future Athletic Trainers' Society, and actively promotes athletic training education in the community. She has become a big proponent and spokesperson for mental health awareness for both student-athletes and athletic training students. Outside of work, her time is spent enjoying the adventures of raising her 2 teenagers, Annamarie and EJ.

Alison R. Snyder Valier, PhD, ATC, FNATA is a Professor for the Post-Professional Athletic Training Program and Doctor of Athletic Training Program at A. T. Still University (ATSU) in Mesa, Arizona. She also serves as the Assistant Director of Research Support through Research, Grants, and Information Technology Systems, as well as a research faculty in the School of Osteopathic Medicine–Arizona, at ATSU.

Dr. Valier received her BA degree in psychology and physical education from Whitman College (Walla Walla, Washington) and her MS in exercise physiology at the University of Toledo (Toledo, Ohio). In addition, she received her PhD in exercise science from the University of Toledo, where she majored in applied physiology and completed a minor in human anatomy. Dr. Valier completed a Post-Doctoral Research Fellowship in Clinical Outcomes Research, with emphasis on the evaluation of patient-reported outcomes instruments and epidemiology, awarded to her by the National Athletic Trainers' Association Research and Education Foundation (NATA REF). Her fellowship has shaped her teaching and research emphasis, with most of her focus on clinical outcomes assessment, patient-reported outcome measures, health-related quality of life, sports injury epidemiology, and quality improvement. She presents and publishes on these topics regularly and is a Fellow of the NATA. Over the years, Dr. Valier has served the profession in many ways, including being a member of the NATA Pronouncements Committee, NATA REF Research Committee, and the Rocky Mountain Athletic Trainers' Association (RMATA) Programming Committee. She also serves as the Co-Chair of the Arizona Athletic Trainers' Association Governmental Affairs Committee and served as the Chair of the Free Communication program for the RMATA for several years. Dr. Valier lives in Gilbert, Arizona, with her husband, Sean, and son, Albert.

PREFACE

The fourth edition of *Special Tests for Orthopedic Examination* was designed to follow our initial goals of providing a simple pocket-sized manual for practical learning purposes. Consistent with previous editions, we updated the content by both removing and adding a few tests. And in keeping with the tradition of enhancing each version, the fourth edition features improvements that we think will be well received. Likely the biggest change that you will notice is the inclusion of a section titled "Evidence" where we have highlighted systematic reviews, meta-analyses, or single articles that have addressed the reliability and/or diagnostic accuracy of the special tests. We've included evidence in this edition as a response to one of the most common requests we received from formal reviews and informal feedback. You will note that some tests have evidence and others do not. Some of the evidence is in support of tests and some is not. The range or spread of some of the diagnostic accuracy values is wide and this may make some readers a little unsure of whether or not to use a particular test. Consistent with previous editions of this text, we don't make the decision on which tests to use for the clinician because there are many considerations that come into play when selecting a test. Further, we purposefully did not exclude tests without evidence to support their effectiveness because clinical discussion has favored their empirical use. Once again, we challenge each of you to come to your own conclusions, and perhaps formulate your own research to support or refute tests with limited or no evidence. While in past editions we have always continued to demonstrate these 3-dimensional tests as best we can in a 2-dimensional format, this edition is accompanied by ancillary material available on the publisher's website depicting videos for each test. The addition of the videos should help clinicians with better understanding the test motion and performing them accurately. It is our hope that you will appreciate this much needed, extremely helpful addition.

SPECIAL TESTS: A KEY CLINICAL SKILL

Webster defines the word "special" as "distinguished by some unusual quality" and "designed for a particular purpose or occasion," and the word "test" as "a critical examination, observation, or evaluation."

In any orthopedic evaluation process, the use of special tests assists to provide critical information leading to, confirming, ruling in, ruling out, and monitoring the status of a particular diagnostic condition. It is no wonder then that in the day of diagnostic imaging and advanced technological interventions clinicians often resort to the basic skills of manual examination for a sense of comfort during the examination process.

As stated in the previous 3 editions of this text, special tests are merely one part of the evaluation process that also relies heavily on history taking, symptoms, diagnostic findings, and other information from the patient, among many other components. Yet in the algorithmic approach to determining what musculoskeletal and/or neurological structures may or may not have been damaged, key special tests often come in handy.

It is important to further elaborate on how we as authors chose to include the specials tests within the book, and how we suggest you use the information to be effective as a clinician. The compilation of the tests in this book reflect a number of ways of thinking. First, tests included are ones that the editors have seen commonly documented and described in numerous orthopedic and sports medicine-related textbooks as well as through clinical practice experiences. Since the first edition of this book, there has been advancement in the study of these tests, however, we still have a long way to go. As you explore the selection of special tests, you will find that some tests have been studied and we know more about their ability to rule in and rule out conditions now than before. You will also find that many tests have not been studied. While we don't know about the reliability, validity, or diagnostic accuracy of these unexamined special tests, they are continually published and taught in curricula and used in clinical practice. Inclusion of these tests may not seem to jive with the current agenda of evidenced-based medicine, yet how can one challenge a clinician who regularly uses a particular special test and has accuracy in diagnostic decision making and treatment intervention that is partially a result of the special test and its findings or lack thereof? Given this fact, we will continue to include unexamined special tests in hope that either one day such tests will have demonstrated validity, reliability, and/or diagnostic accuracy or we as individually talented clinicians within our own rights will come to realize the functionality of these test may not be simply classified as "yes, it works" or "no, it doesn't work." After all, part of evidence-based medicine is also to determine the "how's" and "when's". How do swelling, pain, and range of motion limitations influence the effectiveness of a special test? How does the experience of the examining clinician influence the findings? What about the clinician's hand size, height, setting, and even bedside manner when performing a test? The simple message here is that regardless of how much evidence is reviewed and which way the evidence points, some special tests may or may not work in the hands of different individuals or with different patient presentations. And, the available literature is not exhaustive in considering all of these situations. Once again, in the words of Dr. Joe Gieck, "At first you do what you're taught, and then you do what works."

While it is our belief that each clinician should judge for him- or herself whether there is benefit of using a particular test in a specific clinical circumstance, making informed decisions is important, too. Over the years, different research teams have evaluated many of the tests included in this book, and we feel that it is useful to clinicians to have examples of the available information to help in decision making. Evidence can help inform clinical decisions. So, for the first time, we have included evidence regarding reliability, sensitivity, and specificity of the special tests, where available.

Recall that reliability refers to the reproducibility of the test and is captured with various statistical measures such as the intraclass correlation coefficient, referred to as the ICC, and the Kappa coefficient. Reliability can be computed for multiple scores from one rater, called intrarater reliability, or it can be calculated between more than one rater, called interrater reliability. Reliability values closer to 1 suggest more reliability in the scoring system than values closer to zero. Let's consider the Ober's Test that is used to test for iliotibial band tightness. One study has found that the intrarater reliability of the Ober's Test is .90, which suggests that the test is highly reliable.

Sensitivity and specificity speak to the diagnostic accuracy of measurement or screening tools, including special tests. Sensitivity speaks to our ability to rule out a health condition, such as a ligament tear, whereas specificity helps us rule in a health condition. Values for sensitivity and specificity may be reported differently, but generally are in the range of 0 to 100, with values closer to 100 having greater diagnostic ability than values closer to 0. Let's consider the Anterior Lachman's Test that is used to check for anterior cruciate ligament (ACL) tears. Two recent meta-analyses reported the sensitivity and specificity of the Anterior Lachman's Test. While the reported values from these meta-analyses are slightly different, with sensitivity reported as 81 and 85 and specificity as 81 and 94, the values in either case are, generally speaking, high. The high sensitivity of the Anterior Lachman's Test means that a negative finding could rule out an ACL tear. The high specificity of the Anterior Lachman's Test means that a positive finding could rule in an ACL tear. While there are other values that help with evaluating the diagnostic accuracy of tests, such as likelihood ratios and positive and negative predictive values, we have focused on sensitivity and specificity because they are commonly reported in diagnostic accuracy studies and tend to be constant across multiple samples and populations. Other indices must be customized for the sample of interest, based on the expected prevalence of the condition of interest within the population from which the sample was drawn.

Because this is not meant to be a research text, but instead a quick resource for clinicians, it will be helpful to describe our process for evidence selection and presentation. We could have conducted our search in many ways. After careful thought and consideration, we focused on an approach to find the best type of summary evidence available. Summary evidence, such as from systematic reviews and meta-analyses, typically is considered to have a high level of evidence and is the type of evidence we sought to include in the book. Initially, we searched major search engines, such as PubMed, for key words that included the test name, body part or body region evaluated, and injury. Other key words included special tests, orthopedic tests, provocative tests, sensitivity, specificity, and reliability. Our searching produced numerous articles from which to draw information. Whenever possible, we have reported evidence from systematic reviews and meta-analyses. However, not all special tests have been studied and of those that have been studied, not all have been part of a systematic review or meta-analysis. So, when we didn't find evidence from a systematic review or meta-analysis, we selected a couple single studies and highlighted their findings. Once articles were identified, we pulled basic information about the studies, including any information on reliability, sensitivity, and specificity, and put it into a table for easy viewing. Even though we have included evidence in this edition, it's important to note that editing this text does not render us authorities of special tests, but rather providers of information. As one knows, peer-reviewed manuscripts can be discussed in forums of professionals who do not agree on the interpretation of the manuscript, the statistic used, and sometimes even the accuracy of the conclusions. Determining whether or not a special test referred to in this book should be used by a clinician or not is beyond the goal of this book. It is our belief that each clinician should judge for him- or herself as to whether or not a particular test is found to be useful in certain circumstances within his or her own orthopedic assessment, and we have presented evidence to help in making that judgment.

It is also important to consider where a special test falls in the overall concept of evidence-based practice. Most medical and health care professionals believe that in addition to the actual research-based findings related to a special test, technique, or intervention, there are other important factors that exist that assist in determining what actually constitutes as "good" overall evidence. Specifically, the experience and expertise of an individual clinician, and the perceived and actual value as reported by the patient, both play an integrated role in establishing a final determination. Thus, to reiterate, it is difficult with many of these special tests to simply conclude whether one "works" or "doesn't work."

In summary, the fourth edition was needed and brings some new features for the reader. We've enjoyed putting it together! As always, we remind you that special tests are merely a piece of the puzzle that assist in the evaluation process. While you piece your puzzles together, we hope that this new edition will provide you with a handy tool for problem solving.

—*Jeff G. Konin, PhD, ATC, PT, FACSM, FNATA*
—*Denise Lebsack, PhD, ATC*
—*Alison R. Snyder Valier, PhD, ATC, FNATA*
—*Jerome A. "Jai" Isear, Jr., MS, PT, LAT, ATC*

FOREWORD

It is a special honor for me to write the Foreword to this book for several reasons. First, I have known Dr. Konin for many years professionally, and he has assembled an experienced group of authors who have considerable expertise in the examination of patients with musculoskeletal complaints. Their scholarship and integrity is without reproach.

The second reason is that as an author of this Foreword I am joining distinguished names like Craig Denegar, PhD, PT, ATC, FNATA; Jim Andrews, MD; and Mark Miller, MD! Very flattering.

The third reason is that the physical examination in orthopedic surgery has for a long time been a favorite field of interest for me. What stimulated me to be interested in this topic was that many of the physical examination tests that I was taught as a medical student, as an orthopedic resident, and as a sports medicine fellow simply did not seem to be helpful in clinical practice. For example, like many people I was taught that a Speed's Test was diagnostic of biceps tendon problems, but many of the patients who had a positive test were found to have no biceps tendon pathology at all when an arthroscopy was performed. Many had other pathologies that would explain their "biceps pain." It is now appreciated that anterior shoulder pain can be due to stiffness, arthritis, rotator cuff syndromes, or any number of other pathologies. When scientifically studied, the literature demonstrates that the Speed's Test has largely low sensitivity or specificity for biceps disorders. I still use a Speed's Test just for fun but do not hang my hat on any diagnosis using that test alone. The authors correctly state and demonstrate again in this book that a correct diagnosis starts with a careful history and thorough examination, but one must know how to do the examination first.

Which brings me to what is wonderful about the new format of this book. The authors have not lost the main goal of having a handy guide that defines a specific test and that shows one how to perform the test. It is a great book for the pocket or white coat to refer to at short notice. This applies to every joint from the fingertips to the toes including the spine. As a result, this book still has appeal for anyone who does musculoskeletal medicine, whether novice or experienced in the field.

The second wonderful thing about this book is that the authors updated it with new tests and removed some proven not to be helpful. It is not a static but a dynamic book in that regard. There are new figures in this book and new information; it is not just a rehash of old information. The most important addition in this edition of the book is the inclusion of scientific information about the clinical usefulness of the tests. When teaching students, residents, or anyone else about musculoskeletal exams, I tell them there are 3 levels. The first is to learn what the name of the test is and how to do it. The next is to know the meaning of the test and what is a positive test and what is a negative test. The third level is to know how to interpret the test and how accurate it is in helping to make the diagnosis. This third level is what is exciting about this book because it helps anyone doing these examinations understand why the result may or may not establish a diagnosis. Some tests are great for making a diagnosis and some stink. As the authors say, it is up to each individual to use the tests and to get an impression of what works and what does not work. This book reinforces those impressions with hard data to give the examiner a guide as to whether to trust a test or not.

The musculoskeletal examination is a dynamic skill that does not stay static; our appreciation of what works and what does not work also changes as more examination tests are described and as more tests are studied scientifically. This book now does it all: how to perform and to understand the musculoskeletal examination for the beginner, the "expert," and everyone in between.

—Edward G. McFarland, MD
The Wayne H. Lewis Professor of Shoulder Surgery
Department of Orthopaedic Surgery
The Johns Hopkins University
Baltimore, Maryland

Section

1

Temporomandibular

Guide to Figures

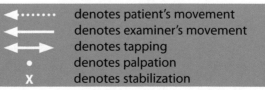

- ◀┈┈┈┈ denotes patient's movement
- ◀─── denotes examiner's movement
- ◀──▶ denotes tapping
- • denotes palpation
- x denotes stabilization

Konin JG, Lebsack D, Snyder Valier AR, Isear JA Jr.
Special Tests for Orthopedic Examination, Fourth Edition (pp 1-6).
© 2016 SLACK Incorporated.

TEMPOROMANDIBULAR

CHVOSTEK'S SIGN

TEST POSITIONING

The subject can either sit or stand.

ACTION

The examiner taps over the masseter muscle and parotid gland (Figure T1-1).

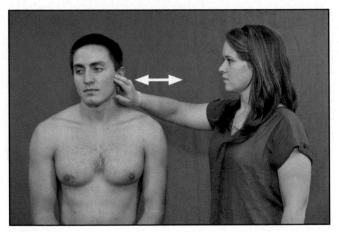

Figure T1-1.

POSITIVE FINDING

Twitching of the facial muscles, especially the masseter, indicates positive findings for facial nerve pathology.

SPECIAL CONSIDERATIONS/COMMENTS

Twitching of the facial muscles may also be a result of low calcium levels in the blood. A positive finding of this nature has also been referred to as a Weiss Sign.

REFERENCES

Hasan ZU, Absamara R, Ahmed M. Chvostek's sign in paediatric practice. *Curr Pediatr Rev.* 2014;10(3):194-197.

Kugelberg E. The mechanism of Chvostek's sign. *AMA Arch Neurol Psychiatry.* 1951;65(4):511-517.

Urbano FL. Signs of hypocalcemia: Chvostek's and Trousseau's signs. *Hosp Physician.* 2000;36(3):43-45.

LOADING TEST

TEST POSITIONING

The subject sits upright in a chair.

ACTION

The examiner places a cotton roll between the molars on the uninvolved side and instructs the subject to bite down forcefully.

POSITIVE FINDING

The reporting of pain on the involved side by the subject indicates a positive finding, which may be reflective of an anteriorly dislocated disk.

SPECIAL CONSIDERATIONS/COMMENTS

The subject may be instructed to chew on the cotton as opposed to forcefully biting down. A positive finding for pain may suggest any number of temporomandibular pathologies.

REFERENCES

Chin LP, Aker FD, Zarrinnia K. The viscoelastic properties of the human temporomandicular joint disk. *J Oral Maxillofac Surg*. 1996;54(3)315-318.

Huddleston Slater JJ, Visscher CM, Lobbezoo F, Naeije M. The intra-articular distance within the TMJ during free and loaded closing movements. *J Dent Res*. 1999;78(12):1815-1820.

Jonsson C, Eckerdal O, Isberg A. Thickness of the articular soft tissue of the temporal component in temporomandibular joints with and without disk displacement. *Oral Surg Med Oral Pathol Oral Radiol Endod*. 1999;87(1):20-26.

Naeije M, Hofman N. Biomechanics of the human temporomandibular joint during chewing. *J Dent Res*. 2003;82(7):528-531.

Nickel JC, Iwasaki LR, Beatty MW, Marx DB. Laboratory stresses and tractional forces on the TMJ disc surface. *J Dent Res*. 2004;83(8):650-654.

Walilko T, Bir C, Godwin W, King A. Relationship between temporomandibular joint dynamics and mouthguards: feasibility of a test method. *Dent Traumatol*. 2004;20(5):255-260.

PALPATION TEST

TEST POSITIONING

The subject sits upright in a chair.

ACTION

The examiner faces the subject and places his or her fifth digits in the subject's ears. The subject is instructed to repeatedly open and close the mouth while the examiner applies pressure in an anterior direction using the pads of the fifth digits (Figures T1-2A and T1-2B).

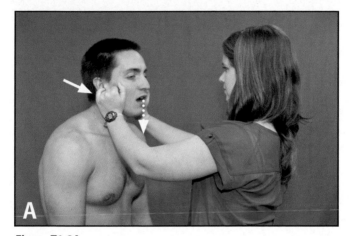

Figure T1-2A.

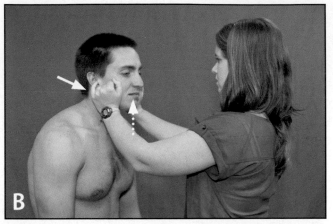

Figure T1-2B.

POSITIVE FINDING

The subject's reporting of pain or discomfort during the opening and closing of the mouth when pressure is applied indicates a positive test. This may be a result of inflammation to the synovium of the temporomandibular joint (TMJ).

SPECIAL CONSIDERATIONS/COMMENTS

The subjective reporting of pain can be a result of any pathology to the TMJ.

REFERENCES

Chase DC, Hendler BH. Spelling relief for TMJ troubles. *Patient Care.* 1988;22(12):158.

Haley DP, Schiffman EL, Lindgren BR, Anderson Q, Andreasen K. The relationship between clinical and MRI findings in patients with unilateral temporomandibular joint pain. *J Am Dent Assoc.* 2001;132(4):476-481.

Huddleston Slater JJ, Lobbezoo F, Van Selms MK, Naeije M. Recognition of internal derangements. *J Oral Rehabil.* 2004;31(9):851-854.

Please see videos on the accompanying website at
www.healio.com/books/specialtestsvideos

Section

2

Cervical Spine

Guide to Figures

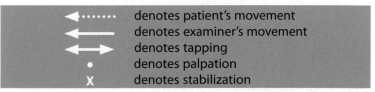

←······· denotes patient's movement
←—— denotes examiner's movement
←→ denotes tapping
• denotes palpation
x denotes stabilization

Konin JG, Lebsack D, Snyder Valier AR, Isear JA Jr.
Special Tests for Orthopedic Examination, Fourth Edition (pp 7-19).
© 2016 SLACK Incorporated.

VERTEBRAL ARTERY TEST

TEST POSITIONING

The subject lies supine, and the examiner sits with both hands supporting the subject's head.

ACTION

Slowly extend, rotate, and laterally flex the subject's cervical spine to each side. Then observe the subject for dizziness, blurred vision, nystagmus, slurred speech, or loss of consciousness (Figure CS2-1). Each position should be held for approximately 30 seconds.

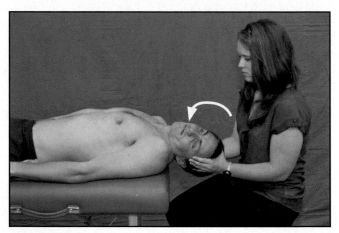

Figure CS2-1.

POSITIVE FINDING

Dizziness, blurred vision, nystagmus, slurred speech, or loss of consciousness are indicative of partial or complete occlusion of the vertebral artery.

SPECIAL CONSIDERATIONS/COMMENTS

The aforementioned signs and symptoms should be considered contraindications for treatments such as traction and joint mobilizations.

REFERENCES

Côté P, Kreitz BG, Cassidy JD, Thiel H. The validity of the extension-rotation test as a clinical screening procedure before neck manipulation: a secondary analysis. *J Manipulative Physiol Ther.* 1996;19(3):159-164.

Licht PB, Christensen HW, Høilund-Carlsen PF. Carotid artery blood flow during premanipulative testing. *J Manipulative Physiol Ther.* 2002;25(9):568-572.

Mitchell J, Keene D, Dyson C, Harvey L, Pruvey C, Phillips R. Is cervical spine rotation, as used in the standard vertebrobasilar insufficiency test, associated with a measureable change in intracranial vertebral artery blood flow? *Man Ther.* 2004;9(4):220-227.

Westaway MD, Stratford P, Symons B. False-negative extension/rotation pre-manipulative screening test on a patient with an atretic and hypoplastic vertebral artery. *Man Ther.* 2003;8(2):120-127.

Zaina C, Grant R, Johnson C, Dansie B, Taylor J, Spyropolous P. The effect of cervical rotation on blood flow in the contralateral vertebral artery. *Man Ther.* 2003;8(2):103-109.

FORAMINAL COMPRESSION TEST (SPURLING)

TEST POSITIONING

With the subject seated comfortably, the examiner rests the volar surface of both hands on top of the subject's head (Figure CS2-2A).

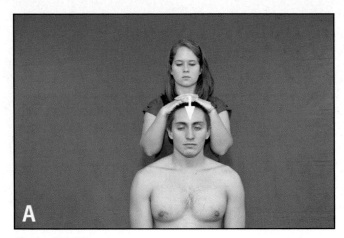

Figure CS2-2A.

ACTION

The examiner applies a downward pressure while the subject laterally flexes the head. The test is repeated with the subject laterally flexing to the opposite side. Lateral flexion may be performed both actively and passively (Figure CS2-2B).

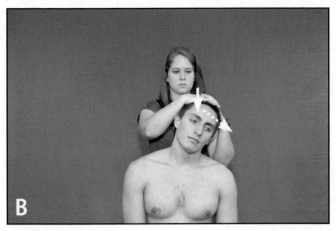

Figure CS2-2B.

POSITIVE FINDING

During the application of compression, a reporting of pain into the upper extremity toward the same side that the head is laterally flexed is positive. This indicates pressure on a nerve root, which can be correlated by the dermatomal distribution of the pain.

SPECIAL CONSIDERATIONS/COMMENTS

Precautions (and possibly avoidance) should be taken with compression of the vertebral area with a subject who has been diagnosed with conditions such as osteoarthritis, rheumatoid arthritis, osteoporosis, and spinal stenosis. The examiner should perform the vertebral artery test as a screen prior to administering this special test.

EVIDENCE

	Rubinstein et al (2007)	Shabat et al (2011)
Study design	Systematic review	Cross-sectional
Conditions evaluated	Cervical radiculopathy	Cervical radiculopathy
Study number	4	
Sample size		257
Reliability	Not evaluated	Not evaluated
Sensitivity	50 to 100	95
Specificity	86 to 100	94

REFERENCES

Dvorák J. Epidemiology, physical examination, and neurodiagnostics. Spine (Phila Pa 1976). 1998;23(24):2663-2672.

Levitz CL, Reilly PJ, Torg JS. The pathomechanics of chronic, recurrent, cervical nerve root neurapraxia. The chronic burner syndrome. Am J Sports Med. 1997;25(1):73-76.

Malanga GA. The diagnosis and treatment of cervical radiculopathy. Med Sci Sports Exerc. 1997;29(7 Suppl):S236-S245.

Rubinstein SM, Pool JJ, van Tulder MW, Riphagen II, de Vet HC. A systematic review of the diagnostic accuracy of provocative tests of the neck for diagnosing cervical radiculopathy. Eur Spine J. 2007;16(3):307-319.

Shabat S, Leitner Y, David R, Folman Y. The correlation between Spurling test and imaging studies in detecting cervical radiculopathy. J Neuroimaging. 2011;22(4):375-378.

Shah KC, Rajshekhar V. Reliability of diagnosis of soft cervical disc prolapse using Spurling's test. Br J Neurosurg. 2005;18(5):480-483.

Spurling RG, Scoville WB. Lateral rupture of the cervical intervertebral disks. Surg Gynecol Obstet. 1944;78:350-358.

Tong HC, Haig AJ, Yamakawa K. The Spurling test and cervical radiculopathy. Spine (Phila Pa 1976). 2002;27(2):156-159.

Uchihara T, Furukawa T, Tsukagoshi H. Compression of brachial plexus as a diagnostic test of cervical cord lesion. Spine (Phila Pa 1976). 1994;19(19):2170-2173.

FORAMINAL DISTRACTION TEST

TEST POSITIONING

With the subject seated, the examiner places one hand under the subject's chin and the other hand around the occiput (Figure CS2-3).

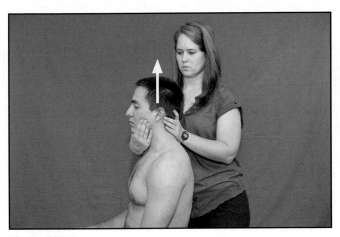

Figure CS2-3.

ACTION

The examiner slowly distracts the subject's head from the trunk while the subject remains in a relaxed position.

POSITIVE FINDING

The finding is positive when existing complaints of pain decrease or disappear during the distraction. This indicates that a nerve root compression may exist while the subject sustains normal posture and/or positioning.

SPECIAL CONSIDERATIONS/COMMENTS

Distraction of the cervical area for the assessment of a nerve root impingement should not be performed on a subject who has vertebral instability. Any increase in pain may indicate muscular and/ or ligamentous damage. The examiner should perform the Vertebral Artery Test as a screen prior to administering this special test.

EVIDENCE

	Wainner and Gill (2000)	Rubinstein et al (2007)
Study design	Literature review	Systematic review
Conditions evaluated	Cervical radiculopathy	Cervical radiculopathy
Study number	2	2
Reliability	Kappa = .5	Not evaluated
Sensitivity	40	44
Specificity	100	90 to 97

REFERENCES

Kruse-Lösler B, Meyer U, Flören C, Joos U. Influence of distraction rates on the temporomandibular joint position and cartilage morphology in a rabbit model of mandibular lengthening. *J Oral Maxillofac Surg.* 2001;59(12):1452-1459.

Rathore S. Use of McKenzie cervical protocol in the treatment of radicular neck pain in a machine operator. *J Can Chiropr Assoc.* 2003;47(4):291-297.

Rubinstein SM, Pool JJ, van Tulder MW, Riphagen II, de Vet HC. A systematic review of the diagnostic accuracy of provocative tests of the neck for diagnosing cervical radiculopathy. *Eur Spine J.* 2007;16(3):307-319.

Wainner RS, Fritz JM, Irrgang JJ, Boninger ML, Delitto A, Allison S. Reliability and diagnostic accuracy of the clinical examination and patient self-report measures for cervical radiculopathy. *Spine (Phila Pa 1976).* 2003;28(1):52-62.

Wainner RS, Gill H. Diagnosis and nonoperative management of cervical radiculopathy. *J Orthop Sports Phys Ther.* 2000;30(12):728-744.

VALSALVA'S MANEUVER

TEST POSITIONING

The subject is seated. The examiner stands next to the subject.

ACTION

The examiner asks the subject to take a deep breath and hold while bearing down, as if having a bowel movement.

POSITIVE FINDING

Increased pain due to increased intrathecal pressure, which may be secondary to a space-occupying lesion, herniated disk, tumor, or osteophyte in the cervical canal, is a positive finding. Pain may be localized or referred to the corresponding dermatome.

SPECIAL CONSIDERATIONS/COMMENTS

The increased pressure may alter venous function and cause dizziness or unconsciousness. The examiner should be prepared to steady the subject.

EVIDENCE

	Wainner et al (2003)
Study design	Diagnostic accuracy
Conditions evaluated	Cervical radiculopathy
Sample size	82
Reliability	Kappa = .69
Sensitivity	22
Specificity	94

REFERENCES

Childs JD. One on one. The impact of the Valsalva maneuver during resistance exercise. *Strength Cond J.* 1999;21(2):54-55.

Dyste KH, Newkirk KM. Pneumomediastinum in a high school football player: a case report. *J Athl Train.* 1998;33(4):362-364.

Folta A, Metzger BL, Therrien B. Preexisting physical activity level and cardiovascular responses across the Valsalva maneuver. *Nurs Res.* 1989;38(3):139-43.

Goldish GD, Quast JE, Blow JJ, Kuskowski MA. Postural effects on intra-abdominal pressure during Valsalva maneuver. *Arch Phys Med Rehabil.* 1994;75(3):324-327.

Kollef MH, Neelon-Kollef RA. Pulmonary embolism associated with the act of defecation. *Heart Lung.* 1991;20(5 Pt 1):451-454.

Lu Z, Metzger BL, Therrien B. Ethnic differences in physiological responses associated with the Valsalva maneuver. *Res Nurs Heath.* 1990;13(1):9-15.

Metzger BL, Therrien B. Effect of position on cardiovascular response during the Valsalva maneuver. *Nurs Res.* 1990;39(4):198-202.

Naliboff BD, Gilmore SL, Rosenthal MJ. Acute autonomic responses to postural change, Valsalva maneuver, and paced breathing in older type II diabetic men. *J Am Geriatr Soc.* 1993;41(6):648-653.

Nornhold P. Decreased cardiac output from Valsalva maneuver. *Nursing.* 1986;16(10):33.

O'Connor P, Sforzo GA, Frye P. Effect of breathing instruction on blood pressure responses during isometric exercise. *Phys Ther.* 1989;69(9):757-761.

Pierce MJ, Weesner CL, Anderson AR, Albohm MJ. Pneumomediastinum in a female track and field athlete: a case report. *J Athl Train.* 1998;33(2):168-170.

Rubinstein SM, Pool JJ, van Tulder MW, Riphagen II, de Vet HC. A systematic review of the diagnostic accuracy of provocative tests of the neck for diagnosing cervical radiculopathy. *Eur Spine J.* 2007;16(3):307-319.

Tentolouris N, Tsapogas P, Papazachos G, Katsilambros N. Corrected QT interval during the Valsalva maneuver in diabetic subjects. *Diabetes.* 2000;49(5):168.

Therrien B. Position modifies carotid artery blood flow velocity during straining. *Res Nurs Health.* 1990;13(2):69-76.

Wainner RS, Fritz JM, Irrgang JJ, Boninger ML, Delitto A, Allison S. Reliability and diagnostic accuracy of the clinical examination and patient self-report measures for cervical radiculopathy. *Spine (Phila Pa 1976).* 2003;28(1):52-62.

SWALLOWING TEST

TEST POSITIONING

The subject is seated. The examiner stands next to the subject.

ACTION

The examiner asks the subject to swallow.

POSITIVE FINDING

Increased pain or difficulty swallowing (dysphagia) caused by anterior cervical spine obstructions, such as vertebral subluxations, osteophyte protrusion, soft tissue swelling, or tumors in the anterior cervical spine region, is a positive finding.

SPECIAL CONSIDERATIONS/COMMENTS

Be certain the subject's head is neutral because swallowing becomes more difficult with the neck extended.

REFERENCES

Hinds NP, Wiles CM. Assessment of swallowing and referral to speech and language therapists in acute stroke. *QJM.* 1998;91(12):829-835.

Ilbay K, Evliyaoglu C, Etus V, Ozkarakas H, Ceylan S. Abnormal bony protuberance of anterior atlas causing dysphagia. A rare congenital anomaly. *Spinal Cord.* 2004;42(2):129-131.

Meng NH, Wang TG, Lien IN. Dysphagia in patients with brainstem stroke: incidence and outcome. *Am J Phys Med Rehabil.* 2000;79(2):170-196.

Srinivas P, George J. Cervical osteoarthropathy: an unusual cause of dysphagia. *Age Ageing.* 1999;28(3):321-322.

Teramoto S, Fukuchi Y. Detection of aspiration and swallowing disorder in older stroke patients: simple swallowing provocation test versus water swallowing test. *Arch Phys Med Rehabil.* 2000;81(11):1517-1519.

Tohara H, Saitoh E, Mays KA, Kuhlemeier K, Palmer JB. Three tests for predicting aspiration without videofluorography. *Dysphagia.* 2003;18(2):126-134.

Winslow CP, Winslow TJ, Wax MK. Dysphonia and dysphagia following the anterior approach to the cervical spine. *Arch Otolaryngol Head Neck Surg.* 2001;127(1):51-55.

Wu MC, Chang YC, Wang TG, Lin LC. Evaluating swallowing dysfunction using a 100-ml water swallowing test. *Dysphagia.* 2004;19(1):43-47.

TINEL'S SIGN

TEST POSITIONING

The subject can sit or lie supine.

ACTION

The examiner gently taps the cervical area near Erb's point, which can be found anterior to the transverse process of C6, approximately 2 cm superior to the location of the clavicle (Figure CS2-4).

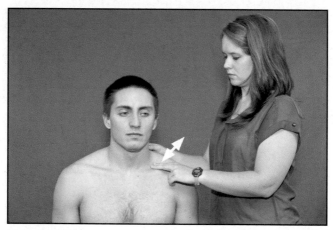

Figure CS2-4.

POSITIVE FINDING

A subjective reporting of a change in sensation to the upper extremity on the ipsilateral side resulting in increased pain or absent/diminished sensation is a positive finding, indicating brachial plexus pathology.

SPECIAL CONSIDERATIONS/COMMENTS

This area is believed to be where the proximal portion of the brachial plexus is most superficial. A positive finding should be combined with a complete cervical nerve root assessment prior to any involved pathology to the brachial plexus.

REFERENCES

Howard M, Lee C, Dellon AL. Documentation of brachial plexus compression (in the thoracic inlet) utilizing provocative neurosensory and muscular testing. *J Reconstr Microsurg.* 2003;19(5):303-312.

Ide M, Ide J, Yamaga M, Takagi K. Symptoms and signs of irritation of the brachial plexus in whiplash injuries. *J Bone Joint Surg Br.* 2001;83(2):226-229.

Please see videos on the accompanying website at
www.healio.com/books/specialtestsvideos

Section
3

Shoulder

Guide to Figures

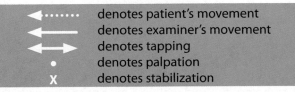

◄········ denotes patient's movement
◄─────── denotes examiner's movement
◄──────► denotes tapping
•   denotes palpation
x   denotes stabilization

Konin JG, Lebsack D, Snyder Valier AR, Isear JA Jr.
Special Tests for Orthopedic Examination, Fourth Edition (pp 21-100).
© 2016 SLACK Incorporated.

EMPTY CAN (SUPRASPINATUS) TEST

TEST POSITIONING

The subject stands with both shoulders abducted to 90 degrees, horizontally adducted 30 degrees, and internally rotated so the subject's thumbs face the floor (Figure S3-1).

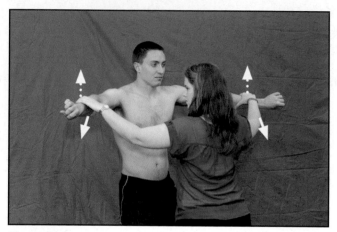

Figure S3-1.

ACTION

The examiner resists the subject's attempts to actively forward elevate both shoulders.

POSITIVE FINDING

Involvement of the supraspinatus muscle and/or tendon is suspected with noted weakness and/or a report of pain.

SPECIAL CONSIDERATIONS/COMMENTS

Although the Empty Can Test is commonly performed with the subject standing, the test may also be performed with the subject seated. Weakness of the supraspinatus muscle may be a result of suprascapular nerve involvement. Reported pain may be indicative of tendinitis and/or impingement.

Evidence

	Hegedus et al (2008)	Hegedus (2012)
Study design	Systematic review	Systematic review
Conditions evaluated	Mixed conditions (eg, impingement syndrome and rotator cuff pathology)	Mixed conditions (eg, supraspinatus pathology, subacromial impingement, rotator cuff pathology)
Study number	1	13
Reliability	Not evaluated	Not evaluated
Sensitivity	44 to 53	19 to 99
Specificity	82 to 90	30 to 100

References

Hegedus EJ. Which physical examination tests provide clinicians with the most value when examining the shoulder? Update of a systematic review with meta-analysis of individual tests. *Br J Sports Med.* 2012;46(14):964-978.

Hegedus EJ, Goode A, Campbell S, et al. Physical examination tests of the shoulder: a systematic review with meta-analysis of individual tests. *Br J Sports Med.* 2008;42(2):80-92; discussion 92.

Holtby R, Razmjou H. Validity of the supraspinatus test as a single clinical test in diagnosing patients with rotator cuff pathology. *J Orthop Sports Phys Ther.* 2004;34(4):194-200.

Itoi E, Kido T, Sano A, Urayama M, Sato K. Which is more useful, the "full can test" or the "empty can test," in detecting the torn supraspinatus tendon? *Am J Sports Med.* 1999;27(1):65-68.

Rowlands LK, Wertsch JJ, Primack SJ, Spreitzer AM, Roberts MM. Kinesiology of the empty can test. *Am J Phys Med Rehabil.* 1995;74(4):302-304.

SHOULDER

YERGASON TEST

TEST POSITIONING

The subject sits with the elbow flexed to 90 degrees and stabilized against the thorax. The forearm is in a pronated position. The examiner places one hand along the subject's forearm and the other hand on the proximal portion of the subject's humerus, near the bicipital groove (Figure S3-2A).

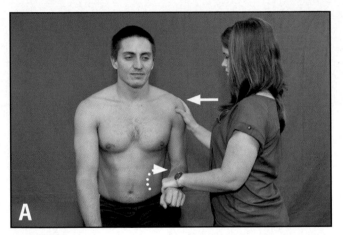

Figure S3-2A.

ACTION

The examiner resists the subject's attempt to actively supinate the forearm and externally rotate the humerus (Figure S3-2B).

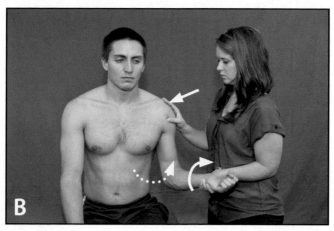

Figure S3-2B.

POSITIVE FINDING

Pain that is reported to exist in the area of the bicipital groove is a positive finding that may indicate bicipital tendinitis.

SPECIAL CONSIDERATIONS/COMMENTS

This is a difficult test to perform. One may be just as accurate to assess bicipital tendinitis by simply palpating the long head of the biceps tendon in the bicipital groove.

EVIDENCE

	Hegedus et al (2008)	Hegedus (2012)
Study design	Systematic review	Meta-analysis
Conditions evaluated	Labral pathology	Biceps tendinopathy
Study number	4	3
Sample size		246
Reliability	Not evaluated	Not evaluated
Sensitivity	12 to 43	12.4
Specificity	79 to 98	95.3

REFERENCES

Caliş M, Akgün K, Birtane M, Karacan I, Caliş H, Tüzün F. Diagnostic values of clinical diagnostic tests in subacromial impingement syndrome. *Ann Rheum Dis.* 2000;59(1):44-47.

Guanche CA, Jones DC. Clinical testing for tears of the glenoid labrum. *Arthroscopy.* 2003;19(5):517-523.

Hegedus EJ. Which physical examination tests provide clinicians with the most value when examining the shoulder? Update of a systematic review with meta-analysis of individual tests. *Br J Sports Med.* 2012;46(14):964-978.

Hegedus EJ, Goode A, Campbell S, et al. Physical examination tests of the shoulder: a systematic review with meta-analysis of individual tests. *Br J Sports Med.* 2008;42(2):80-92; discussion 92.

Yergason RM. Supination sign. *J Bone Joint Surg Am.* 1931;13:160.

SPEED'S TEST

TEST POSITIONING

The subject is seated or standing. The involved shoulder is flexed to 90 degrees, the elbow is fully extended, and the forearm is supinated. The examiner places one hand along the volar aspect of the subject's forearm and the other hand on the proximal aspect of the subject's humerus near the area of the bicipital groove (Figure S3-3).

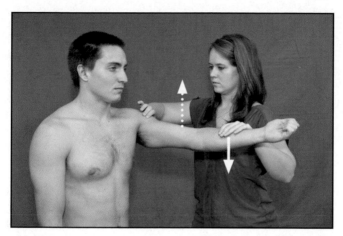

Figure S3-3.

ACTION

The examiner resists the subject's attempt to actively flex the humerus forward.

POSITIVE FINDING

Tenderness and/or pain in the bicipital groove is a positive finding that may suggest bicipital tendinitis.

SPECIAL CONSIDERATIONS/COMMENTS

The examiner should carefully watch that the forearm is supinated and that the subject does not use accessory muscles to mask any existing weakness. Although this test is primarily used to evaluate the biceps tendon, Speed's Test has also been used to evaluate superior labrum anterior to posterior (SLAP) lesions and subacromial impingement.

EVIDENCE

	Hegedus et al (2008)	Hegedus (2012)
Study design	Meta-analysis	Meta-analysis
Conditions evaluated	Labral pathology (eg, SLAP tear)	Labral pathology (eg, biceps tendinopathy)
Study number	4	4
Sample size		327
Reliability	Not evaluated	Not evaluated
Sensitivity	32	20
Specificity	61	78

REFERENCES

Caliş M, Akgün K, Birtane M, Karacan I, Caliş H, Tüzün F. Diagnostic values of clinical diagnostic tests in subacromial impingement syndrome. *Ann Rheum Dis*. 2000;59(1):44-47.

Clarnette RG, Miniaci A. Clinical exam of the shoulder. *Med Sci Sports Exerc*. 1998;30(4 Suppl):S1-S6.

Guanche CA, Jones DC. Clinical testing for tears of the glenoid labrum. *Arthroscopy*. 2003;19(5):517-523.

Hegedus EJ. Which physical examination tests provide clinicians with the most value when examining the shoulder? Update of a systematic review with meta-analysis of individual tests. *Br J Sports Med*. 2012;46(14):964-978.

Hegedus EJ, Goode A, Campbell S, et al. Physical examination tests of the shoulder: a systematic review with meta-analysis of individual tests. *Br J Sports Med*. 2008;42(2):80-92; discussion 92.

Mason JM. Shoulder injury: water polo 584. *Med Sci Sports Exerc*. 1997;29(5):101.

Russ DW. In-season management of shoulder pain in a collegiate swimmer: a team approach. *J Orthop Sports Phys Ther*. 1998;27(5):371-376.

Ludington's Sign

Test Positioning

The subject sits or stands while the examiner stands directly behind the subject. The subject interlocks the fingers and places them on the superior/posterior aspect of the head.

Action

The examiner palpates the long head of the biceps tendon bilaterally while the subject contracts both the left and right biceps brachii muscles simultaneously (Figure S3-4).

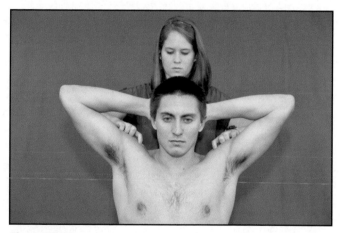

Figure S3-4.

Positive Finding

Increased pain is indicative of a biceps brachii long head tendinitis. Decreased tension of the tendon with palpation may indicate an inability or apprehension of the biceps brachii to contract forcefully.

SPECIAL CONSIDERATIONS/COMMENTS

The subject should be sure to stabilize the humeral head during the contraction and allow for the hands to push into the stabilized humeral head. No tension may be the result of a biceps brachii long head rupture.

REFERENCE

Ludington NA. Rupture of the long head of the biceps flexor cubiti muscle. *Ann Surg.* 1923:77(3);358-363.

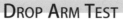

Drop Arm Test

Test Positioning

The subject is seated or standing.

Action

The examiner passively abducts the subject's involved arm to 90 degrees and then instructs the subject to slowly lower the arm to the side (Figures S3-5A and S3-5B).

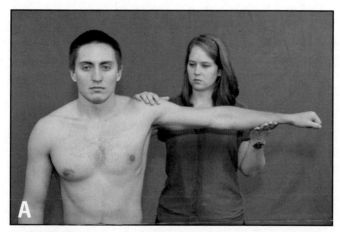

Figure S3-5A.

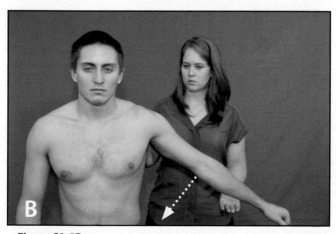

Figure S3-5B.

SHOULDER

POSITIVE FINDING

The subject is unable to slowly return the arm to the side and/or has significant pain when attempting to perform the task. This is indicative of rotator cuff pathology.

SPECIAL CONSIDERATIONS/COMMENTS

If the examiner suspects rotator cuff pathology prior to performing the test, he or she should prepare to rapidly assist the subject in the event that the subject does experience an inability to control the adduction movement of the arm.

EVIDENCE

	Hegedus et al (2008)	Hegedus (2012)
Study design	Systematic review	Systematic review
Conditions evaluated	Impingement and rotator cuff tendinopathies	Impingement and rotator cuff tendinopathies
Study number	3	3
Reliability	Not evaluated	Not evaluated
Sensitivity	8 to 35	24 to 74
Specificity	88 to 100	66 to 93

REFERENCES

Caliş M, Akgün K, Birtane M, Karacan I, Caliş H, Tüzün F. Diagnostic values of clinical diagnostic tests in subacromial impingement syndrome. *Ann Rheum Dis.* 2000;59(1):44-47.

Hegedus EJ. Which physical examination tests provide clinicians with the most value when examining the shoulder? Update of a systematic review with meta-analysis of individual tests. *Br J Sports Med.* 2012;46(14):964-978.

Hegedus EJ, Goode A, Campbell S, et al. Physical examination tests of the shoulder: a systematic review with meta-analysis of individual tests. *Br J Sports Med.* 2008;42(2):80-92; discussion 92.

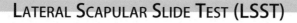

LATERAL SCAPULAR SLIDE TEST (LSST)

TEST POSITIONING

Position 1: The subject stands with arms relaxed at the sides.

Position 2: The subject stands with hands on the hips and shoulders in 10 degrees of extension.

Position 3: The subject stands with shoulders abducted to 90 degrees and maximally internally rotated.

ACTION

Position 1: The examiner measures the distance from the inferior angle of the scapula (involved side) to the spinous process of the thoracic vertebra in the same horizontal plane (this vertebra will be used as the reference vertebra for all 3 positions) (Figure S3-6A). This is repeated on the uninvolved side. The difference between sides is used for the objective assessment.

Position 2: Repeat the same action as in Position 1 (Figure S3-6B).

Position 3: Repeat the same action as in Position 1 (Figure S3-6C).

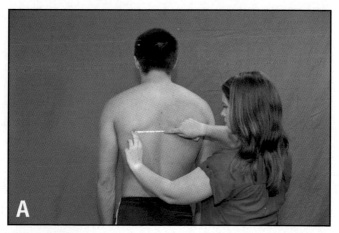

Figure S3-6A.

SHOULDER

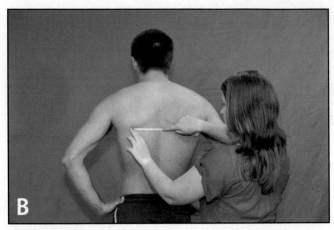

Figure S3-6B.

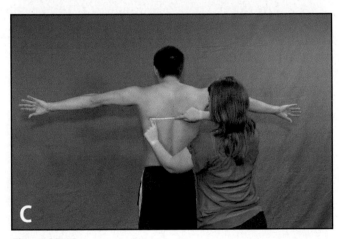

Figure S3-6C.

POSITIVE FINDING

A side-to-side difference of >1.5 cm is considered a positive LSST, indicating scapular asymmetry secondary to weakness of the scapular stabilizers.

SPECIAL CONSIDERATIONS/COMMENTS

The reliability, sensitivity, and specificity of this test in assessing/predicting shoulder dysfunction have been questioned. Because this test is considered a semi-dynamic test only, it may not accurately assess the stabilizing strength of the scapular muscles. It may more accurately assess general asymmetries, leading the clinician to further assess the underlying cause of these asymmetries (eg, motor control, or lack thereof; inflexibilities; thoracic spine/postural deviations).

EVIDENCE

	Shadmehr et al (2014)
Study design	Cross-sectional, repeated measures
Conditions evaluated	Scapular positioning
Sample size	30
Reliability	Position 1: intraclass correlation (ICC) = .87 Position 2: ICC = .77
Sensitivity	Not evaluated
Specificity	Not evaluated

REFERENCES

Crotty NM, Smith J. Alterations in scapular position with fatigue: a study in swimmers. *Clin J Sports Med.* 2000;10(4):251-258.

Kibler WB. The role of the scapula in athletic shoulder function. *Am J Sports Med.* 1998;26(2):325-337.

Koslow PA, Prosser LA, Strony GA, Suchecki SL, Mattingly GE. Specificity of the lateral scapular slide test in asymptomatic competitive athletes. *J Orthop Sports Phys Ther.* 2003;33(6):331-336.

Odom CJ, Taylor AB, Hurd CE, Denegar CR. Measurement of scapular asymmetry and assessment of shoulder dysfunction using the lateral scapular slide test: a reliability and validity study. *Phys Ther.* 2001;81(2):799-809.

Shadmehr A, Azarsa MH, Jalaie S. Inter- and intrarater reliability of modified lateral scapular slide test in healthy athletic men. *Biomed Res Int.* 2014;2014:384149.

SHOULDER

APLEY'S SCRATCH TEST

TEST POSITIONING

The subject may sit or stand. The examiner stands next to the subject.

ACTION 1

The subject is instructed to take one hand and touch the opposite shoulder. Repeat with the other hand to the opposite side (Figure S3-7A).

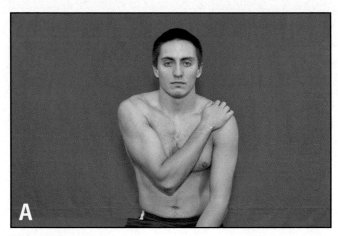

Figure S3-7A.

POSITIVE FINDING 1

Asymmetrical results from side to side are positive. The inability to touch the opposite shoulder is indicative of limited glenohumeral adduction, internal rotation, and horizontal flexion. Limits in scapular protraction may also produce asymmetrical results.

ACTION 2

The subject is then instructed to place the arm overhead and reach behind the neck as if scratching the upper back. Repeat with the opposite side (Figure S3-7B).

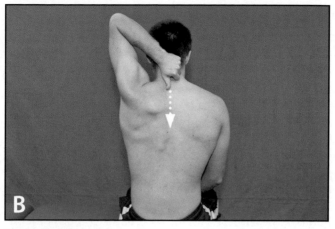

Figure S3-7B.

POSITIVE FINDING 2

Asymmetrical results from side to side are positive. Decreased motion on one side is indicative of limited glenohumeral abduction and external rotation, and scapular upward rotation and elevation.

ACTION 3

The subject is then instructed to place the hand in the small of the back and reach upward as far as possible. Repeat with the opposite side (Figure S3-7C).

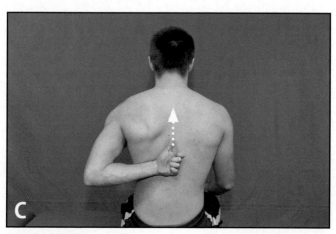

Figure S3-7C.

Positive Finding 3

Asymmetrical results from side to side are positive. Decreased motion on one side is indicative of limited glenohumeral adduction and internal rotation, and scapular retraction and downward rotation.

Special Considerations/Comments

Each of these movements is an active test of the functional mobility of the shoulder. Care should be taken to isolate movements that are restricted. It is not uncommon for a subject to have slightly greater restriction on the dominant shoulder as compared to the nondominant shoulder due to increased muscle mass on the dominant side. For the latter 2 test components, the tester can correlate the thumb of the subject with the level of the spinous process being reached for assessment comparisons over time. The examiner should also assess scapular asymmetries that may be present with glenohumeral motion.

References

Buchberger DJ. The prevalence of subscapularis dysfunction in a baseball population. *Med Sci Sports Exerc.* 1999;31(5):S262.

Endo K, Yukata K, Yasui N. Influence of age on scapulo-thoracic orientation. *Clin Biomech (Bristol, Avon).* 2004;19(10):1009-1013.

CROSS-OVER IMPINGEMENT TEST

TEST POSITIONING

The subject sits. The examiner stands with one hand on the posterior aspect of the subject's shoulder to stabilize the trunk and the other hand grasping the subject's elbow on the test arm.

ACTION

With the subject's trunk stabilized, the examiner passively and maximally horizontally adducts the test shoulder (Figure S3-8).

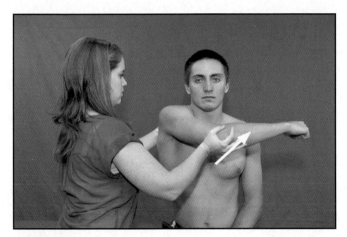

Figure S3-8.

POSITIVE FINDING

Superior shoulder pain is indicative of acromioclavicular joint pathology. Anterior shoulder pain is indicative of subscapularis, supraspinatus, and/or biceps long head pathology. Posterior shoulder pain is indicative of infraspinatus, teres minor, and/or posterior capsule pathology.

SPECIAL CONSIDERATIONS

Although the test is commonly performed with the subject seated, the test may also be performed with the subject in a supine position.

EVIDENCE

	Hegedus et al (2008)	Hegedus (2012)
Study design	Systematic review	Systematic review
Conditions evaluated	Impingement and rotator cuff pathologies	Supraspinatus and rotator cuff tendinopathies; acromioclavicular osteoarthritis
Study number	2	3
Reliability	Not evaluated	Not evaluated
Sensitivity	23 to 82	22 to 77
Specificity	28 to 82	61 to 79

REFERENCES

Berg EE, Ciullo JV. A clinical test for superior glenoid labral or superior labrum anterior-posterior (SLAP) lesions. *Clin J Sport Med.* 1998;8(2):121-123.

Caliş M, Akgün K, Birtane M, Karacan I, Caliş H, Tüzün F. Diagnostic values of clinical diagnostic tests in subacromial impingement syndrome. *Ann Rheum Dis.* 2000;59(1):44-47.

Hegedus EJ. Which physical examination tests provide clinicians with the most value when examining the shoulder? Update of a systematic review with meta-analysis of individual tests. *Br J Sports Med.* 2012;46(14):964-978.

Hegedus EJ, Goode A, Campbell S, et al. Physical examination tests of the shoulder: a systematic review with meta-analysis of individual tests. *Br J Sports Med.* 2008;42(2):80-92; discussion 92.

POSTERIOR IMPINGEMENT TEST

TEST POSITIONING

The subject lies supine on a table with the test shoulder placed in 90 to 110 degrees of abduction and 10 to 15 degrees of extension. The test elbow is flexed to 90 degrees. The examiner sits or stands. The examiner's distal hand grasps the subject's wrist and hand, and the proximal hand grasps the subject's elbow (Figure S3-9A).

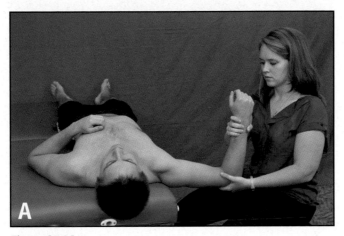

Figure S3-9A.

ACTION

The examiner slowly rotates the subject's shoulder into maximal external rotation (Figure S3-9B).

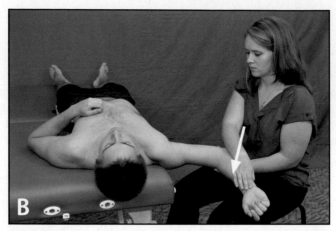

Figure S3-9B.

POSITIVE FINDING

Reproduction of the subject's pain in the posterior aspect of the shoulder is indicative of rotator cuff and/or posterior labral pathology.

SPECIAL CONSIDERATIONS/COMMENTS

This test should not be confused with the Apprehension Test or Relocation Test. The Posterior Impingement Test will reproduce posterior shoulder pain, whereas the Apprehension and Relocation Tests will reproduce anterior shoulder pain and apprehension. Clinically, the Posterior Impingement Test will often correlate highly with the subjective complaints of posterior/superior shoulder pain during the late cocking to acceleration phase of throwing or swinging in the overhand athlete.

EVIDENCE

	Meister et al (2004)
Study design	Diagnostic accuracy
Conditions evaluated	Rotator cuff and labral pathologies
Sample size	69
Reliability	Not evaluated
Sensitivity	76
Specificity	85

REFERENCES

Meister K, Buckley B, Batts J. The posterior impingement sign: diagnosis of rotator cuff and posterior labral tears secondary to internal impingement in overhand athletes. *Am J Orthop (Belle Mead NJ)*. 2004;33(8):412-415.

Walch G, Boileau P, Noel E, Donell ST. Impingement of the deep surface of the supraspinatus tendon on the posterosuperior glenoid rim: an arthroscopic study. *J Shoulder Elbow Surg.* 1992;1(5):238-245.

NEER IMPINGEMENT TEST

TEST POSITIONING

The subject sits or stands with both upper extremities relaxed. The examiner stands with one hand on the scapula (posteriorly) and the other hand grasping near the subject's elbow (anteriorly).

ACTION

With the subject's scapula stabilized, the examiner passively and maximally forward-flexes the test shoulder (Figure S3-10).

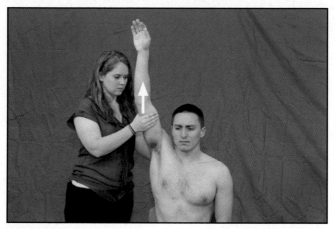

Figure S3-10.

POSITIVE FINDING

Shoulder pain and apprehension are indicative of shoulder impingement, particularly of the supraspinatus and biceps long head tendons.

SPECIAL CONSIDERATIONS/COMMENTS

A false-positive test may be elicited if the subject has limited forward flexion to the extent that anatomical impingement is not the limiting factor.

EVIDENCE

	Hegedus et al (2008)	Hegedus (2012)
Study design	Meta-analysis	Meta-analysis
Conditions evaluated	Subacromial impingement	Mixed conditions (eg, subacromial impingement, biceps tendinopathy)
Study number	4	7
Sample size		946
Reliability	Not evaluated	Not evaluated
Sensitivity	79	72
Specificity	53	60

SHOULDER

REFERENCES

Caliş M, Akgün K, Birtane M, Karacan I, Caliş H, Tüzün F. Diagnostic values of clinical diagnostic tests in subacromial impingement syndrome. *Ann Rheum Dis.* 2000;59(1):44-47.

Cavallo RJ, Speer KP. Shoulder instability and impingement in throwing athletes. *Med Sci Sports Exerc.* 1998;30(4 Suppl):S18-S25.

Hegedus EJ. Which physical examination tests provide clinicians with the most value when examining the shoulder? Update of a systematic review with meta-analysis of individual tests. *Br J Sports Med.* 2012;46(14):964-978.

Hegedus EJ, Goode A, Campbell S, et al. Physical examination tests of the shoulder: a systematic review with meta-analysis of individual tests. *Br J Sports Med.* 2008;42(2):80-92; discussion 92.

Kirkley A, Litchfield RB, Jackowski DM, Lo IK. The use of the impingement test as a predictor of outcome following subacromial decompression for rotator cuff tendinosis. *Arthroscopy.* 2002;18(1):8-15.

Neer CS II. Anterior acromioplasty for the chronic impingement syndrome in the shoulder: a preliminary report. *J Bone Joint Surg Am.* 1972;54(1):41-50.

Zaslav KR. Internal rotation resistance strength test: a new diagnostic test to differentiate intra-articular pathology from outlet (Neer) impingement syndrome in the shoulder. *J Shoulder Elbow Surg.* 2001;10(1)23-27.

HAWKINS-KENNEDY IMPINGEMENT TEST

TEST POSITIONING

The subject sits or stands with both upper extremities relaxed. The examiner stands with one hand grasping the subject's elbow and the other hand grasping the subject's wrist, both on the test arm.

ACTION

The examiner flexes the elbow to 90 degrees, forward-flexes the shoulder to 90 degrees, and then internally rotates the subject's test shoulder (Figure S3-11).

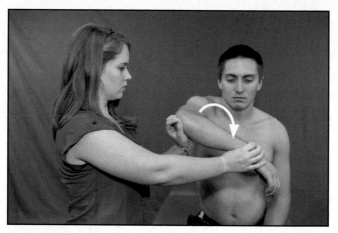

Figure S3-11.

POSITIVE FINDING

Shoulder pain and apprehension are indicative of shoulder impingement, particularly of the supraspinatus tendon.

SPECIAL CONSIDERATIONS/COMMENTS

This test tends to be the most sensitive for assessing subacromial impingement.

EVIDENCE

	Hegedus et al (2008)	Hegedus (2012)
Study design	Meta-analysis	Meta-analysis
Conditions evaluated	Subacromial impingement	Subacromial impingement
Study number	4	7
Sample size		944
Reliability	Not evaluated	Not evaluated
Sensitivity	79	80
Specificity	59	56

REFERENCES

Caliş M, Akgün K, Birtane M, Karacan I, Caliş H, Tüzün F. Diagnostic values of clinical diagnostic tests in subacromial impingement syndrome. *Ann Rheum Dis.* 2000;59(1):44-47.

De Wilde L, Plasschaert F, Berghs B, Van Hoecke M, Verstraete K, Verdonk R. Quantified measurement of subacromial impingement. *J Shoulder Elbow Surg.* 2003;12(4):346-349.

Hawkins RJ, Kennedy JC. Impingement syndrome in athletics. *Am J Sports Med.* 1980;8(3):151-158.

Hegedus EJ. Which physical examination tests provide clinicians with the most value when examining the shoulder? Update of a systematic review with meta-analysis of individual tests. *Br J Sports Med.* 2012;46(14):964-978.

Hegedus EJ, Goode A, Campbell S, et al. Physical examination tests of the shoulder: a systematic review with meta-analysis of individual tests. *Br J Sports Med.* 2008;42(2):80-92; discussion 92.

Kirkley A, Litchfield RB, Jackowski DM, Lo IK. The use of the impingement test as a predictor of outcome following subacromial decompression for rotator cuff tendinosis. *Arthroscopy.* 2002;18(1):8-15.

MacDonald PB, Clark P, Sutherland K. An analysis of the diagnostic accuracy of the Hawkins and Neer subacromial impingement signs. *J Shoulder Elbow Surg.* 2000;9(4):299-301.

Struhl S. Anterior internal impingement: an arthroscopic observation. *Arthroscopy.* 2002;18(1):2-7.

Valadie AL III, Jobe CM, Pink MM, Ekman EF, Jobe FW. Anatomy of provocative tests for impingement syndrome of the shoulder. *J Shoulder Elbow Surg.* 2000;9(1):36-46.

STERNOCLAVICULAR (SC) JOINT STRESS TEST

TEST POSITIONING

The subject sits with the involved arm relaxed at the side. The examiner stands in front of the subject, placing one hand on the proximal end of the subject's clavicle and the other hand on the spine of the scapula (Figure S3-12).

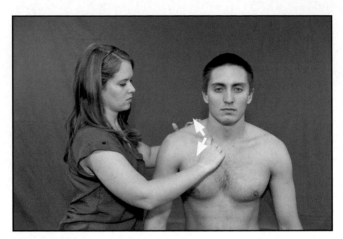

Figure S3-12.

ACTION

The examiner applies gentle inferior and posterior pressure on the clavicle, noting any movement at the SC joint.

POSITIVE FINDING

Pain and/or movement of the clavicle indicates an SC ligament sprain, possibly involving the costoclavicular ligament.

SPECIAL CONSIDERATIONS/COMMENTS

This test should not be performed if there is obvious SC joint deformity. Caution should also be used if an injury to the trachea region is suspected in addition to SC pathology.

ACROMIOCLAVICULAR (AC) JOINT DISTRACTION TEST

TEST POSITIONING

The subject sits with the involved arm relaxed at the side and the elbow flexed to 90 degrees. The examiner stands on the involved side and holds the subject's arm near the elbow crease with one hand. The examiner's other hand is placed over the involved AC joint (Figure S3-13).

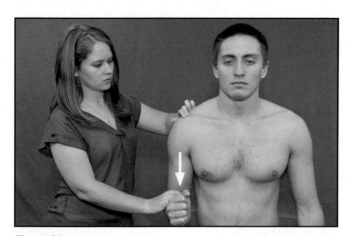

Figure S3-13.

ACTION

The examiner applies gentle downward pressure on the arm, noting any movement at the AC joint.

POSITIVE FINDING

Pain and/or movement of the scapula inferior to the clavicle is positive, indicating AC and/or coracoclavicular ligament sprains.

SPECIAL CONSIDERATIONS/COMMENTS

This test should not be performed if any obvious AC joint deformity exists.

REFERENCE

Chronopoulus E, Kim TK, Park HB, Ashenbrenner D, McFarland EG. Diagnostic value of physical tests for isolated chronic AC lesions. *Am J Sports Med.* 2004;32(3):655-661.

ACROMIOCLAVICULAR (AC) JOINT COMPRESSION TEST (SHEAR)

TEST POSITIONING

The subject sits with the involved arm relaxed at the side. The examiner stands on the involved side, placing one hand on the subject's clavicle and the other hand on the spine of the scapula (Figure S3-14).

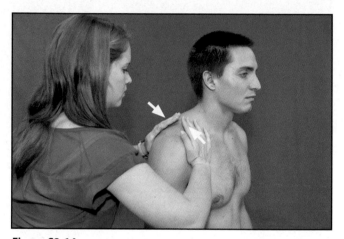

Figure S3-14.

ACTION

The examiner gently squeezes the hands together, noting any movement at the AC joint.

POSITIVE FINDING

Pain and/or movement of the clavicle is a positive indication of an AC and/or coracoclavicular ligament sprain.

SPECIAL CONSIDERATIONS/COMMENTS

This test should not be performed if there is obvious AC joint deformity.

REFERENCES

Chronopoulus E, Kim TK, Park HB, Ashenbrenner D, McFarland EG. Diagnostic value of physical tests for isolated chronic AC lesions. *Am J Sports Med.* 2004;32(3):655-661.

Lee MP. Diagnostic values of tests for acromioclavicular joint pain: a case report. *J Hand Ther.* 2004;17(4):427-428.

O'Brien SJ, Pagnani MJ, Fealy S, McGlynn SR, Wilson JB. The active compression test: a new and effective test for diagnosing labral tears and acromioclavicular joint abnormality. *Am J Sports Med.* 1998;26(5):610-613.

PIANO KEY SIGN

TEST POSITIONING

The subject sits with the involved limb relaxed at the side or stands facing the examiner.

ACTION

The examiner applies downward pressure to the subject's distal clavicle in an inferior direction (Figure S3-15).

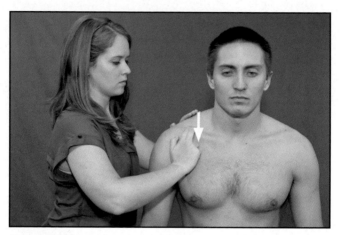

Figure S3-15.

POSITIVE FINDING

The examiner is able to use inferior pressure to depress the clavicle into its normal resting position and subsequently watch the clavicle elevate again once the pressure is removed. This finding is indicative of the instability of the AC joint on the involved side.

SPECIAL CONSIDERATIONS/COMMENTS

The examiner should always use a bilateral comparison when assessing the range of elevation and depression of the involved clavicle. Significant clavicular elevation may also indicate coracoclavicular joint involvement.

APPREHENSION TEST (ANTERIOR)

TEST POSITIONING

The subject lies supine on a table.

ACTION

With the subject's involved shoulder in 90 degrees of abduction and the elbow in 90 degrees of flexion, the examiner slowly externally rotates the shoulder (Figure S3-16).

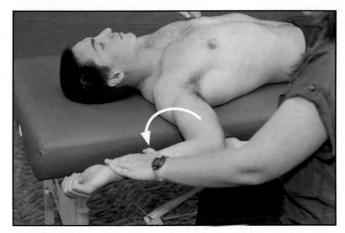

Figure S3-16.

POSITIVE FINDING

A positive finding for this test can be interpreted if the subject looks apprehensive or expresses feelings of apprehension toward further movement in the externally rotated direction. This test is used to mimic the positioning and movement of an anterior dislocation of the glenohumeral joint, thus recreating a subject's episode of instability.

SPECIAL CONSIDERATIONS/COMMENTS

Simple indication or reporting of apprehension to a movement does not necessarily indicate a dislocation of the glenohumeral joint.

EVIDENCE

	Hegedus et al (2008)	Hegedus (2012)
Study design	Systematic review	Meta-analysis
Conditions evaluated	Instability	Mixed conditions (eg, SLAP tear and instability)
Study number	2	2
Sample size		409
Reliability	Not evaluated	Not evaluated
Sensitivity	50 to 72	66
Specificity	56 to 99	95

REFERENCES

Gagey OJ, Gagey N. The hyperabduction test. *J Bone Joint Surg Br.* 2001;83(1):69-74.

Guanche CA, Jones DC. Clinical testing for tears of the glenoid labrum. *Arthroscopy.* 2003;19(5):517-523.

Hegedus EJ. Which physical examination tests provide clinicians with the most value when examining the shoulder? Update of a systematic review with meta-analysis of individual tests. *Br J Sports Med.* 2012;46(14):964-978.

Hegedus EJ, Goode A, Campbell S, et al. Physical examination tests of the shoulder: a systematic review with meta-analysis of individual tests. *Br J Sports Med.* 2008;42(2):80-92; discussion 92.

Kirkley A, Nonweiller B, Lo IKY, Woolfrey M. Validation of the apprehension relocation and surprise tests in the diagnosis of anterior shoulder instability. *J Bone Joint Surg Br.* 1997;79B(Suppl 1):75.

Lo IK, Nonweiler B, Woolfrey M, Litchfield R, Kirkley A. An evaluation of the apprehension, relocation and surprise tests for anterior shoulder instability. *Am J Sports Med.* 2004;32(2):301-307.

Mahaffey BL, Smith PA. Shoulder instability in youth athletes. *Am Fam Physician.* 1999;59(10);2773-2782; 2787.

Wintzell G. Larsson H, Larsson S. The Bankart and Hill-Sachs lesion detected in the apprehension test position by the use of open MRI and intravenous contrast in the unstable shoulder. *J Bone Joint Surg Br.* 1997:79-B(2S):254.

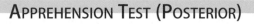

APPREHENSION TEST (POSTERIOR)

TEST POSITIONING

The subject lies supine on a table. The examiner grasps the subject's elbow with one hand and stabilizes the ipsilateral and involved shoulder with the other hand.

ACTION

The examiner places the subject's involved shoulder in a position of 90 degrees of flexion and internal rotation while applying a posterior force through the long axis of the humerus (Figure S3-17).

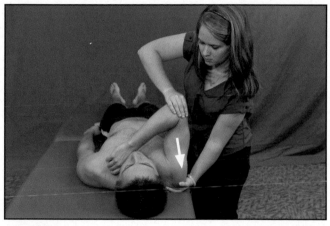

Figure S3-17.

POSITIVE FINDING

A positive finding for this test can be interpreted if the subject looks apprehensive or expresses feelings of apprehension toward further movement in the posterior direction. This test is used to mimic the positioning and movement of a posterior dislocation of the glenohumeral joint, thus recreating a subject's episode of instability.

SPECIAL CONSIDERATIONS/COMMENTS

Simple indication or reporting of apprehension to a movement does not necessarily indicate a dislocation of the glenohumeral joint.

EVIDENCE

	Hegedus (2012)
Study design	Systematic review
Conditions evaluated	Instability
Study number	1
Reliability	Not evaluated
Sensitivity	19
Specificity	99

REFERENCES

Cavallo RJ, Speer KP. Shoulder instability and impingement in throwing athletes. *Med Sci Sports Exerc.* 1998;30(4):18-25.

Hegedus EJ. Which physical examination tests provide clinicians with the most value when examining the shoulder? Update of a systematic review with meta-analysis of individual tests. *Br J Sports Med.* 2012;46(14):964-978.

Tzannes A, Paxinos A, Callanan M, Murrell GA. An assessment of the inter-examiner reliability of tests for shoulder instability. *J Shoulder Elbow Surg.* 2004;13(1):18-23.

SULCUS SIGN

TEST POSITIONING

The subject sits with the forearms and hands resting in the lap. The examiner stands with the proximal hand grasping the subject's scapula (superiorly) and the distal hand grasping the subject's elbow (Figure S3-18).

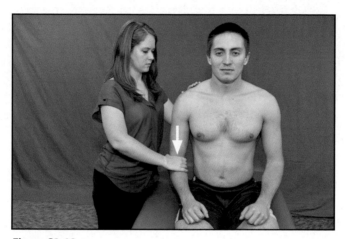

Figure S3-18.

ACTION

With the scapula stabilized, the examiner applies an inferior (distraction) force with the distal hand.

POSITIVE FINDING

Excessive inferior humeral head translation with a visible and/or palpable "step-off" or "sulcus" deformity immediately inferior to the acromion (laterally) is indicative of inferior and/or multidirectional instability.

SPECIAL CONSIDERATIONS/COMMENTS

A positive sulcus sign at rest may indicate excessive capsular stretching. This may also be accompanied by a neurological stretch to structures of the brachial plexus.

EVIDENCE

	Tzannes et al (2004)	Nakagawa et al (2005)
Study design	Reliability	Randomized controlled trial
Conditions evaluated	Instability	Labral pathology
Sample size	13	54
Reliability	ICC = .60	Not evaluated
Sensitivity	Not evaluated	17
Specificity	Not evaluated	93

REFERENCES

Cole BJ, Rodeo SA, O'Brien SJ, et al. The anatomy and histology of the rotator interval capsule of the shoulder. *Clin Orthop Relat Res.* 2001;1(390):129-137.

Nakagawa S, Yoneda M, Hayashida K, Obata M, Fukushima S, Miyazaki Y. Forced shoulder abduction and elbow flexion test: a new simple clinical test to detect superior labral injury in the throwing shoulder. *Arthroscopy.* 2005;21(11):1290-1295.

Tzannes A, Paxinos A, Callanan M, Murrell GA. An assessment of the inter-examiner reliability of tests for shoulder instability. *J Shoulder Elbow Surg.* 2004;13(1):18-23.

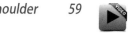

ANTERIOR DRAWER TEST

TEST POSITIONING

The subject lies supine with the glenohumeral joint positioned at the edge of the table. The examiner stands next to the involved shoulder, placing one hand around the humerus below the surgical neck. The other hand stabilizes the scapula by placing the fingers behind the subject on the spine of the scapula and the thumb over the coracoid process (Figure S3-19).

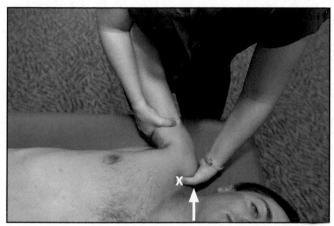

Figure S3-19. Note: Stabilize at the coracoid process and the spine of the scapula.

ACTION

The subject must remain relaxed while the examiner passively abducts the glenohumeral joint 70 to 80 degrees, forward-flexes 0 to 10 degrees, and externally rotates 0 to 10 degrees. While stabilizing the scapula, the examiner firmly glides the head of the humerus anteriorly and applies slight distraction to the glenohumeral joint.

POSITIVE FINDING

Increased anterior translation of the humeral head relative to the scapula/glenoid fossa may be indicative of anterior instability. The subject may exhibit apprehension if the test is positive. A bilateral comparison should be used for a more accurate assessment.

EVIDENCE

	Munro and Healy (2009)	Hegedus et al (2008)	Hegedus (2012)
Study design	Systematic review	Systematic review	Meta-analysis
Conditions evaluated	SLAP lesions	Labral integrity	Labral integrity, biceps tendinopathy
Study number	3	4	4
Sample size			831
Reliability	Not evaluated	Not evaluated	Not evaluated
Sensitivity	5 to 78	5 to 78	17
Specificity	82 to 93	82 to 93	86

REFERENCES

Hegedus EJ. Which physical examination tests provide clinicians with the most value when examining the shoulder? Update of a systematic review with meta-analysis of individual tests. *Br J Sports Med.* 2012;46(14):964-978.

Hegedus EJ, Goode A, Campbell S, et al. Physical examination tests of the shoulder: a systematic review with meta-analysis of individual tests. *Br J Sports Med.* 2008;42(2):80-92; discussion 92.

McQuade KJ, Murthi AM. Anterior glenohumeral force/translation behavior with and without rotator cuff contraction during clinical stability testing. *Clin Biomech (Bristol, Avon).* 2004;19(1):10-15.

McQuade KJ, Shelley I, Cvitkovic J. Patterns of stiffness during clinical examination of the glenohumeral joint. *Clin Biomech (Bristol, Avon).* 1999;14(9):620-627.

Munro W, Healy R. The validity and accuracy of clinical tests used to detect labral pathology of the shoulder—a systematic review. *Man Ther.* 2009;14(2):119-130.

Wang Y, Wang H, Dong S, et al. Clinical study on traumatic anterior instability of shoulder [article in Chinese]. *Zhonghua Wai Ke Za Zhi.* 1998;36(10):588-590.

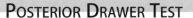
Posterior Drawer Test

Test Positioning

The subject lies supine. The examiner stands next to the involved shoulder, holds the subject's arm at the elbow, passively abducts the shoulder to 30 to 70 degrees, and horizontally flexes the shoulder 20 to 30 degrees. The subject's elbow is flexed in a relaxed position. The examiner stabilizes the scapula by placing the other hand posterior to the shoulder joint capsule with the thumb over the coracoid process (Figure S3-20).

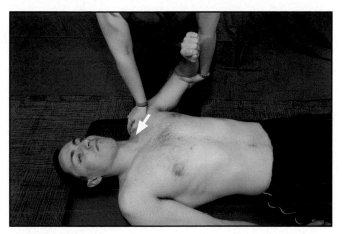

Figure S3-20.

Action

While stabilizing the scapula, the examiner applies downward pressure, pushing the humeral head posteriorly. The examiner notes any posterior movement of the humeral head.

Positive Finding

Increased posterior instability of the humeral head relative to the scapula/glenoid fossa may be indicative of posterior instability. The subject may exhibit apprehension if the test is positive.

SPECIAL CONSIDERATIONS/COMMENTS

A bilateral comparison should be used for a more accurate assessment.

REFERENCES

Emery RJ, Mullaji AB. Glenohumeral joint instability in normal adolescents. Incidence and significance. *J Bone Joint Surg Br.* 1991;73(3):406-408.

McQuade KJ, Shelley I, Cvitkovic J. Patterns of stiffness during clinical examination of the glenohumeral joint. *Clin Biomech (Bristol, Avon).* 1999;14(9):620-627.

JOBE RELOCATION TEST

TEST POSITIONING

The subject lies supine with the test shoulder in 90 degrees of abduction and full external rotation. The examiner stands with the distal hand grasping the subject's wrist and hand. The examiner's proximal hand is placed over the subject's humeral head (anteriorly) (Figure S3-21).

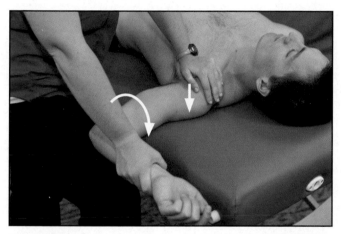

Figure S3-21.

ACTION

The examiner applies a posterior force to the humeral head, while the examiner externally rotates the subject's humerus.

POSITIVE FINDING

A reduction of pain and apprehension, and commonly an increase in shoulder external rotation, are indicative of anterior instability.

SPECIAL CONSIDERATIONS/COMMENTS

This test should be performed immediately following the apprehension test. Pain associated with the Jobe Relocation Test that follows a positive Anterior Apprehension Test may be associated with any number of pathologies not limited to anterior instability. However, if pain is seen with an Anterior Apprehension Test and subsides with a subsequent Jobe Relocation Test, it is quite possible that any pain was in fact associated with a greater than normal anterior gliding of the humeral head.

EVIDENCE

	Tzannes et al (2004)	Hegedus et al (2008)	Hegedus (2012)
Study design	Reliability	Systematic review	Meta-analysis
Conditions evaluated	Symptomatic shoulder patients	Instability	Instability
Study number		3	3
Sample size	13		509
Reliability	ICC = .31 to .71	Not evaluated	Not evaluated
Sensitivity	Not evaluated	30 to 81	65
Specificity	Not evaluated	44 to 99	90

REFERENCES

Hamner DL, Pink MM, Jobe FW. A modification of the relocation test: arthroscopic findings associated with a positive test. *J Shoulder Elbow Surg.* 2000;9(4):263-267.

Hegedus EJ. Which physical examination tests provide clinicians with the most value when examining the shoulder? Update of a systematic review with meta-analysis of individual tests. *Br J Sports Med.* 2012;46(14):964-978.

Hegedus EJ, Goode A, Campbell S, et al. Physical examination tests of the shoulder: a systematic review with meta-analysis of individual tests. *Br J Sports Med.* 2008;42(2):80-92; discussion 92.

Kölbel R. A modification of the relocation test: arthroscopic findings associated with a positive test. *J Shoulder Elbow Surg.* 2001;10(5):497-498.

Lo IK, Nonweiler B, Woolfrey M, Litchfield R, Kirkley A. An evaluation of the apprehension, relocation and surprise tests for anterior shoulder instability. *Am J Sports Med.* 2004;32(2):301-307.

Tzannes A, Paxinos A, Callanan M, Murrell GA. An assessment of the inter-examiner reliability of tests for shoulder instability. *J Shoulder Elbow Surg.* 2004;13(1):18-23.

SHOULDER

SURPRISE TEST (ACTIVE RELEASE TEST)

TEST POSITIONING

The subject lies supine with the test shoulder in 90 degrees of abduction and full external rotation. The examiner stands with the distal hand grasping the subject's wrist and hand. The examiner's proximal hand is placed over the subject's humeral head (anteriorly) (Figure S3-22A).

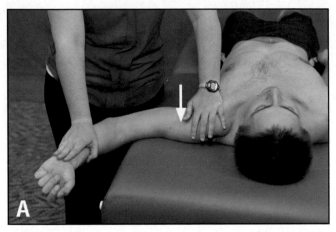

Figure S3-22A.

ACTION

The examiner applies a posterior force to the humeral head while externally rotating the subject's humerus. Then, the examiner quickly removes the proximal hand from the humeral head (Figure S3-22B).

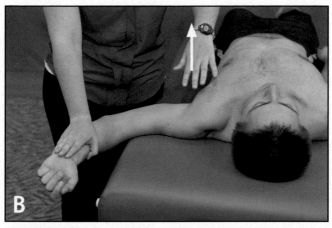

Figure S3-22B.

POSITIVE FINDING

A sudden return of symptoms that were elicited from the Apprehension Test is indicative of anterior instability.

SPECIAL CONSIDERATIONS/COMMENTS

The Surprise Test is merely an extension of the Relocation Test and should therefore be performed immediately following the Apprehension and Relocation Tests, respectively. If the subject demonstrates severe apprehension and instability symptoms with the Apprehension Test, the Surprise Test should not be performed so as not to traumatize (or lose rapport with) the subject.

EVIDENCE

	Hegedus et al (2008)	Hegedus (2012)
Study design	Systematic review	Meta-analysis
Conditions evaluated	Instability	Instability
Study number	2	2
Sample size		128
Reliability	Not evaluated	Not evaluated
Sensitivity	64 to 92	82
Specificity	89 to 99	86

REFERENCES

Hegedus EJ. Which physical examination tests provide clinicians with the most value when examining the shoulder? Update of a systematic review with meta-analysis of individual tests. *Br J Sports Med.* 2012;46(14):964-978.

Hegedus EJ, Goode A, Campbell S, et al. Physical examination tests of the shoulder: a systematic review with meta-analysis of individual tests. *Br J Sports Med.* 2008;42(2):80-92; discussion 92.

Lo IK, Nonweiler B, Woolfrey M, Litchfield R, Kirkley A. An evaluation of the apprehension, relocation and surprise tests for anterior shoulder instability. *Am J Sport Med.* 2004;32(2):301-307.

Tzannes A, Paxinos A, Callanan M, Murrell GA. An assessment of the inter-examiner reliability of tests for shoulder instability. *J Shoulder Elbow Surg.* 2004;13(1):18-23.

FEAGIN TEST

TEST POSITIONING

The subject stands with the involved arm abducted to 70 to 90 degrees. The elbow is extended and allowed to rest on the examiner's shoulder. The examiner stands to the side of the subject and clasps his or her hands together around the upper and middle thirds of the humerus.

ACTION

The examiner attempts to glide the humerus in an anterior and inferior direction (Figure S3-23).

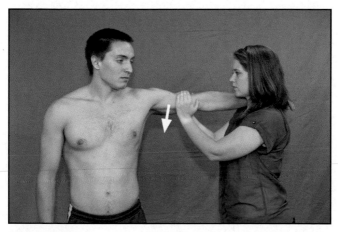

Figure S3-23.

POSITIVE FINDING

Excessive gliding of the humerus (as compared to the noninvolved side) may be indicative of anterior and/or inferior glenohumeral instability.

SHOULDER

SPECIAL CONSIDERATIONS/COMMENTS

The subject may appear to be apprehensive when performing this test. If so, the examiner can conclude only that the test is not sensitive enough to assess instability unless the examiner is able to judge accessory motion compared to the noninvolved side. Apprehension alone cannot be used to predict glenohumeral instability.

REFERENCE

Brenneke SL, Reid J, Ching RP, Wheeler DL. Glenohumeral kinematics and capsulo-ligamentous strain resulting from laxity exams. *Clin Biomech (Bristol, Avon)*. 2000;15(10):735-742.

LOAD AND SHIFT TEST

TEST POSITIONING

The subject sits with no upper trunk stabilization and the involved arm resting at the side. The examiner stands slightly behind the subject while stabilizing the clavicle and scapula with one hand. With the other hand, the examiner grasps the subject's humeral head with the thumb posteriorly. The examiner's remaining fingers are located anteriorly (Figure S3-24).

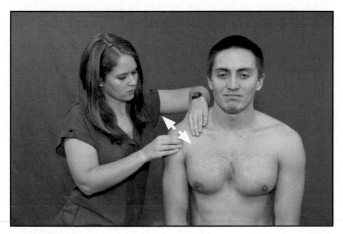

Figure S3-24.

ACTION

The examiner places an axial load along the shaft of the humerus (load) in an attempt to compress the humeral head into the glenoid fossa. With the load applied, the examiner translates the humeral head, first anteriorly (shift) and then posteriorly (shift).

POSITIVE FINDING

An anterior or posterior translation of the humeral head greater than 25% of the diameter of the humeral head when a load is applied is considered to be a positive test. The test should be repeated bilaterally for comparative findings.

SPECIAL CONSIDERATIONS/COMMENTS

Translation between 25% and 50% has been described as being a grade I positive test. Greater than 50% translation associated with a subsequent reduction of the humeral head is considered grade II, whereas the same amount of translation without reduction is recognized as grade III and the most serious type of a shift.

EVIDENCE

	Tzannes et al (2004)
Study design	Reliability
Conditions evaluated	Instability
Sample size	13
Reliability	ICC = .68 to .79
Sensitivity	Not evaluated
Specificity	Not evaluated

REFERENCES

Burkart A, Debski RE, Musahl V, McMahon PJ. Glenohumeral translations are only partially restored after repair of a simulated type II superior labral lesion. *Am J Sports Med*. 2003;31(1):56-63.

Cavallo RJ, Speer KP. Shoulder instability and impingement in throwing athletes. *Med Sci Sports Exerc*. 1998;30(4):18-25.

Fitzpatrick MJ, Tibone JE, Grossman M, McGarry MH, Lee TQ. Development of cadaveric models of a thrower's shoulder. *J Shoulder Elbow Surg*. 2005;14(1 Suppl S):49S-57S.

McMahon PJ, Burkart A, Musahl V, Debski RE. Glenohumeral translations are increased after a type II superior labrum anterior-posterior lesion: a cadaveric study of severity of passive stabilizer injury. *J Shoulder Elbow Surg*. 2004;13(1):39-44.

Tzannes A, Paxinos A, Callanan M, Murrell GA. An assessment of the inter-examiner reliability of tests for shoulder instability. *J Shoulder Elbow Surg*. 2004;13(1):18-23.

SHOULDER

GRIND TEST

TEST POSITIONING

The subject lies supine on a table with the shoulder abducted to 90 degrees and the elbow flexed to 90 degrees on the involved side. The examiner grasps the subject's elbow with one hand and the subject's proximal humerus with the other hand (Figure S3-25).

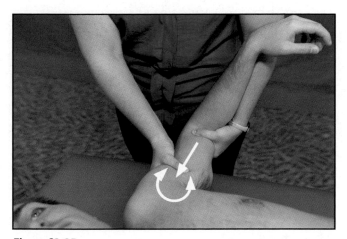

Figure S3-25.

ACTION

The examiner applies compression to the glenoid labrum while attempting to rotate the humeral head 360 degrees around the surface of the glenoid fossa.

POSITIVE FINDING

A positive finding of a grinding or clunking sensation may be indicative of a glenoid labrum tear to the specific location that is being compressed.

SPECIAL CONSIDERATIONS/COMMENTS

This test should be performed carefully because the application of excessive pressure combined with rotation may further damage the glenoid labrum.

CLUNK TEST

TEST POSITIONING

The subject lies supine on a table. The examiner places one hand on the posterior aspect of the subject's humeral head and the other hand proximal to the subject's elbow joint along the distal humerus (Figure S3-26A).

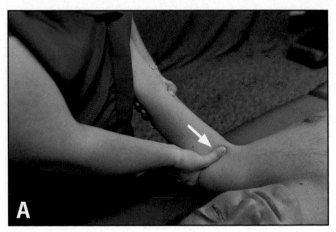

Figure S3-26A.

ACTION

The examiner passively abducts and externally rotates the subject's arm overhead and applies an anterior force to the humerus. (The examiner may also choose to internally rotate the humerus at the same time the anterior force is being applied.) The examiner then circumducts the humeral head around the glenoid labrum (Figure S3-26B).

SHOULDER

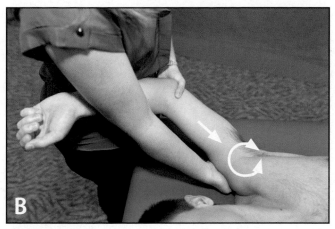

Figure S3-26B.

POSITIVE FINDING

A positive finding of a grinding or clunking sensation may be indicative of a glenoid labrum tear.

SPECIAL CONSIDERATIONS/COMMENTS

The subject may appear to have a positive test or even show apprehension in this position if an underlying anterior and/or inferior instability of the glenohumeral joint exists. This test is most appropriate for assessing superior labral tears because the inferior portion of the labrum is not in contact with the humeral head while the humerus is positioned in full abduction and external rotation. Because of the nature of this anatomical positioning, it is possible to experience a false-negative test if the subject has an inferior labral tear.

SHOULDER

EVIDENCE

	Hegedus et al (2008)
Study design	Systematic review
Conditions evaluated	Labral pathologies
Study number	1
Reliability	Not evaluated
Sensitivity	44
Specificity	68

REFERENCES

Feinstein WK, Lichtman DM. Recognizing and treating midcarpal instability. *Sports Med Arthrosc.* 1998;6(4):270-277.

Hegedus EJ, Goode A, Campbell S, et al. Physical examination tests of the shoulder: a systematic review with meta-analysis of individual tests. *Br J Sports Med.* 2008;42(2):80-92; discussion 92.

Kim SH, Park JC, Park JS, Oh I. Painful jerk test: a predictor of success in nonoperative treatment of painful inferior instability of the shoulder. *Am J Sports Med.* 2004;32(8):1849-1855.

CRANK TEST

TEST POSITIONING

With the subject standing, the examiner places the distal hand on the subject's elbow and the proximal hand on the subject's proximal humerus and then passively elevates the subject's shoulder to 160 degrees in the scapular plane.

ACTION

With the distal hand, the examiner applies a load along the long axis of the humerus while the proximal hand externally (Figure S3-27A) and internally (Figure S3-27B) rotates the humerus.

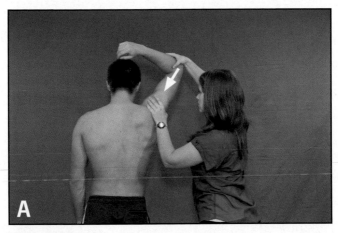

Figure S3-27A.

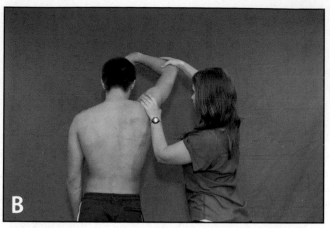

Figure S3-27B.

POSITIVE FINDING

Pain and/or clicking are indicative of glenoid labral pathology.

SPECIAL CONSIDERATIONS/COMMENTS

This test can also be performed in the supine position should apprehension or muscle guarding be a concern in the standing position. Like most tests for labral pathology, the sensitivity of this test is questionable.

EVIDENCE

	Hegedus et al (2008)	Hegedus (2012)
Study design	Systematic review	Meta-analysis
Conditions evaluated	Labral pathologies	Labral pathologies
Study number	5	4
Sample size		282
Reliability	Not evaluated	Not evaluated
Sensitivity	13 to 81	34
Specificity	67 to 88	75

REFERENCES

Guanche CA, Jones DC. Clinical testing for tears of the glenoid labrum. *Arthroscopy.* 2003;19(5):517-523.

Hegedus EJ. Which physical examination tests provide clinicians with the most value when examining the shoulder? Update of a systematic review with meta-analysis of individual tests. *Br J Sports Med.* 2012;46(14):964-978.

Hegedus EJ, Goode A, Campbell S, et al. Physical examination tests of the shoulder: a systematic review with meta-analysis of individual tests. *Br J Sports Med.* 2008;42(2):80-92; discussion 92.

Liu SH, Henry MH, Nuccion SL. A prospective evaluation of a new physical examination in predicting glenoid labral tears. *Am J Sport Med.* 1996;24(6):721-725.

Parentis MA, Mohr KJ, ElAttrache NS. Disorders of the superior labrum: review and treatment guidelines. *Clin Orthop Relat Res.* 2002;(400):77-87.

O'BRIEN TEST (ACTIVE COMPRESSION)

TEST POSITIONING

The subject sits or stands with the test shoulder in 90 degrees of forward flexion, 30 to 45 degrees of horizontal adduction, and maximal internal rotation. The examiner stands with one hand grasping the subject's test wrist (medially) (Figure S3-28A).

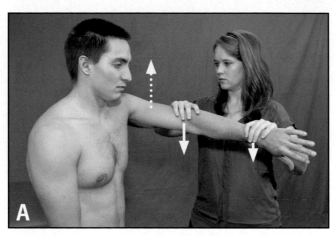

Figure S3-28A.

ACTION

The subject horizontally adducts and flexes the test shoulder against the examiner's manual resistance. The test is then repeated with the subject's arm in an externally rotated position (Figure S3-28B).

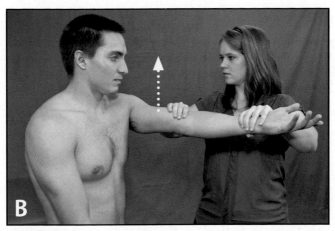

Figure S3-28B.

POSITIVE FINDING

Pain and/or popping that is present in the internally rotated position but absent in the externally rotated position is indicative of a SLAP lesion.

SPECIAL CONSIDERATIONS/COMMENTS

The O'Brien Test is considered to be the most accurate test for assessing SLAP lesions; however, the sensitivity of this and other SLAP lesion tests are questionable. To more closely simulate the eccentric traction associated with the mechanism of injury related to SLAP lesions, the examiner may wish to slowly move the subject's arm from a flexed to an extended position while resisting horizontal adduction and shoulder flexion.

EVIDENCE

	Hegedus et al (2008)	Hegedus (2012)
Study design	Systematic review	Meta-analysis
Conditions evaluated	SLAP lesion	SLAP lesion
Study number	6	6
Sample size		782
Reliability	Not evaluated	Not evaluated
Sensitivity	47 to 99	67
Specificity	11 to 98	37

REFERENCES

Guanche CA, Jones DC. Clinical testing for tears of the glenoid labrum. *Arthroscopy.* 2003;19(5):517-523.

Hegedus EJ. Which physical examination tests provide clinicians with the most value when examining the shoulder? Update of a systematic review with meta-analysis of individual tests. *Br J Sports Med.* 2012;46(14):964-978.

Hegedus EJ, Goode A, Campbell S, et al. Physical examination tests of the shoulder: a systematic review with meta-analysis of individual tests. *Br J Sports Med.* 2008;42(2):80-92; discussion 92.

McFarland EG, Kim TK, Savino RM. Clinical assessment of three common tests for superior labral anterior-posterior lesions. *Am J Sports Med.* 2002;30(6):810-815.

O'Brien SJ, Pagnani MJ, Fealy S, McGlynn SR, Wilson JB. The active compression test: a new and effective test for diagnosing labral tears and acromioclavicular joint abnormality. *Am J Sports Med.* 1998;26(5):610-613.

Parentis MA, Jobe CM, Pink MM, Jobe FW. An anatomic evaluation of the active compression test. *J Shoulder Elbow Surg.* 2004;13(4):410-416.

Stetson WB, Templin K. The crank test, the O'Brien test, and routine magnetic resonance imaging scans in the diagnosis of labral tears. *Am J Sports Med.* 2002;30(6):806-809.

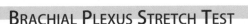

BRACHIAL PLEXUS STRETCH TEST

TEST POSITIONING

The subject sits. The examiner stands next to or behind the subject and places one hand on the side of the subject's head and the other hand on the shoulder of the same side.

ACTION

The examiner laterally flexes the subject's head while applying gentle downward pressure on the shoulder (Figure S3-29).

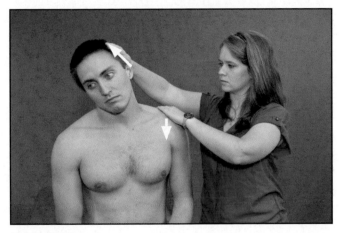

Figure S3-29.

POSITIVE FINDING

Pain that radiates into the subject's arm opposite to the laterally flexed neck indicates a positive finding.

SPECIAL CONSIDERATIONS/COMMENTS

If pain is in the neck on the side toward lateral flexion, a pinched nerve or facet joint impingement may exist. This test should not be performed if a cervical fracture or dislocation is suspected.

REFERENCES

Balster SM, Jull GA. Upper trapezius muscle activity during the brachial plexus tension test in asymptomatic subjects. *Man Ther.* 1997;2(3):144-149.

Mackinnon SE. Pathophysiology of nerve compression. *Hand Clin.* 2002;18(2):231-234.

ADSON'S MANEUVER

TEST POSITIONING

The subject sits or stands. The examiner stands with fingers over the radial artery (distally) (Figure S3-30A).

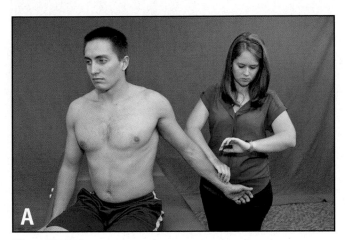

Figure S3-30A.

ACTION

The examiner externally rotates and extends the subject's test arm while palpating the radial pulse. The subject then extends and rotates the neck toward the test arm and takes a deep breath (Figure S3-30B).

SHOULDER

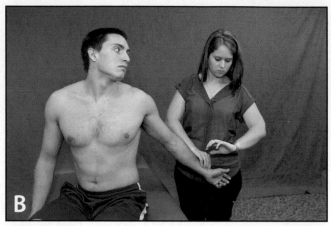

Figure S3-30B.

POSITIVE FINDING

A diminished or absent radial pulse is indicative of thoracic outlet syndrome, secondary to compression of the subclavian artery by the scalene muscles.

SPECIAL CONSIDERATIONS/COMMENTS

This test assesses vascular structures only and has a high incidence (> 50%) of false-positive findings. The examiner should record the rate and rhythm of the pulse as reduced or altered, as opposed to one that is completely diminished.

EVIDENCE

	Plewa and Delinger (1998)	Nord et al (2008)
Study design	Cross-sectional	Cross-sectional
Conditions evaluated	Thoracic outlet syndrome	Thoracic outlet syndrome
Sample size	53	86
Reliability	Not evaluated	Not evaluated
Sensitivity	Not evaluated	Not evaluated
Specificity	89 to 100	80

REFERENCES

Nord KM, Kapoor P, Fisher J, et al. False positive rate of thoracic outlet syndrome diagnostic maneuvers. *Electromyogr Clin Neurophysiol.* 2008;48(2):67-74.

Plewa MC, Delinger M. The false-positive rate of thoracic outlet syndrome shoulder maneuvers in healthy subjects. *Acad Emerg Med.* 1998;5(4):337-342.

Rayan GM, Jensen C. Thoracic outlet syndrome: provocative examination maneuvers in a typical population. *J Shoulder Elbow Surg.* 1995;4(2):113-117.

ALLEN'S TEST

TEST POSITIONING

The subject sits or stands with the test shoulder in 90 degrees of abduction and external rotation, and the elbow in 90 degrees of flexion. The examiner stands with fingers over the radial artery (distally).

ACTION

The subject rotates the neck away from the test arm while the examiner palpates the radial pulse (Figure S3-31).

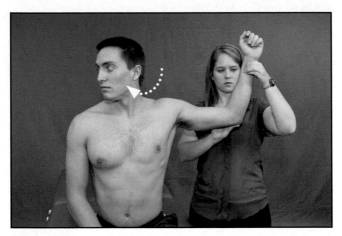

Figure S3-31.

POSITIVE FINDING

A diminished or absent radial pulse is indicative of thoracic outlet syndrome.

SPECIAL CONSIDERATIONS/COMMENTS

This test assesses vascular structures only and has a high incidence (> 50%) of false-positive findings. The examiner should record the rate and rhythm of the pulse as reduced or altered, as opposed to one that is completely diminished.

REFERENCES

Fessler RD, Wakhloo AK, Lanzino G, Guterman LR, Hopkins LN. Transradial approach for vertebral artery stenting: technical case report. *Neurosurgery.* 2000;46(6):1524-1528; discussion 1527-1528.

Owens JC, Blaney LF, Roos DB. Thoracic outlet syndrome. *Bull Soc Int Chir.* 1966;25(5):547-555.

SHOULDER

ROOS TEST (ELEVATED ARM STRESS TEST)

TEST POSITIONING

The subject sits or stands with both shoulders in 90 degrees of abduction and external rotation, and the elbows in 90 degrees of flexion.

ACTION

The subject rapidly opens and closes both hands for 3 minutes (Figures S3-32A and S3-32B).

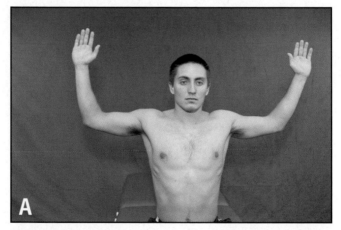

Figure S3-32A.

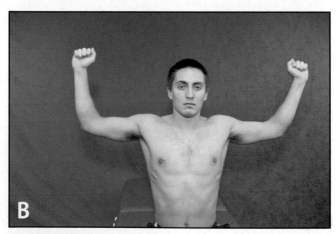

Figure S3-32B.

POSITIVE FINDING

The inability to maintain the test position, diminished motor function of the hands, pain, and/or loss of sensation in the upper extremities are indicative of thoracic outlet syndrome secondary to neurovascular compromise.

SPECIAL CONSIDERATIONS/COMMENTS

This test evaluates both neural and vascular structures and is considered to be the most accurate clinical test for assessing thoracic outlet syndrome. An examiner may find muscle fatigue present when performing the Roos Test for an otherwise healthy population and should therefore use caution when documenting such findings with potential pathologically involved subjects.

EVIDENCE

	Plewa and Delinger (1998)	Nord et al (2008)
Study design	Cross-sectional	Cross-sectional
Conditions evaluated	Thoracic outlet syndrome	Thoracic outlet syndrome
Sample size	53	86
Reliability	Not evaluated	Not evaluated
Sensitivity	Not evaluated	Not evaluated
Specificity	38 to 79	70

REFERENCES

Howard M, Lee C, Dellon AL. Documentation of brachial plexus compression (in the thoracic inlet) utilizing provocative neurosensory and muscular testing. *J Reconstr Microsurg.* 2003;19(5):303-312.

Nord KM, Kapoor P, Fisher J, et al. False positive rate of thoracic outlet syndrome diagnostic maneuvers. *Electromyogr Clin Neurophysiol.* 2008;48(2):67-74.

Owens JC, Blaney LF, Roos DB. Thoracic outlet syndrome. *Bull Soc Int Chir.* 1966;25(5):547-555.

SHOULDER

Plewa MC, Delinger M. The false-positive rate of thoracic outlet syndrome shoulder maneuvers in healthy subjects. *Acad Emerg Med.* 1998;5(4):337-342.

Roos DB. Congenital anomalies associated with thoracic outlet syndrome. Anatomy, symptoms, diagnosis, and treatment. *Am J Surg.* 1976;132(6):771-778.

Roos DB. Experience with first rib resection for thoracic outlet syndrome. *Ann Surg.* 1971;173(3):429-442.

Roos DB. Historical perspectives and anatomic considerations. Thoracic outlet syndrome. *Semin Thorac Cardiovasc Surg.* 1996;8(2):183-189.

Roos DB. Pathophysiology of congenital anomalies in thoracic outlet syndrome. *Acta Chir Belg.* 1980;79(5):353-361.

Roos DB. Thoracic outlet syndrome. *Rocky Mt Med J.* 1967;64(2):49-55.

Roos DB. Transaxillary approach for first rib resection to relieve thoracic outlet syndrome. *Ann Surg.* 1966;163(3):354-358.

Roos DB, Owens JC. Thoracic outlet syndrome. *Arch Surg.* 1966;93(1):71-74.

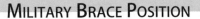

MILITARY BRACE POSITION

TEST POSITIONING

The subject stands in the anatomical position.

ACTION

The examiner stands behind the subject and unilaterally assesses the radial pulse. The subject's same arm is then passively extended and abducted to 30 degrees by the examiner while the subject simultaneously hyperextends the head and neck (Figure S3-33).

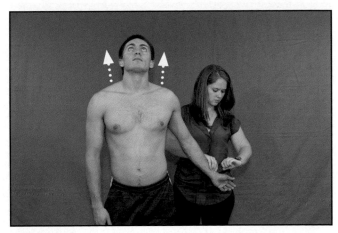

Figure S3-33.

POSITIVE FINDING

A diminished or absent radial pulse may indicate potential thoracic outlet syndrome.

SPECIAL CONSIDERATIONS/COMMENTS

The examiner should assess rate and rhythm of the pulse and note any changes. This assessment should be compared bilaterally. This test is also called the Costoclavicular Syndrome Test, as it is believed a positive finding may be related to a compression of the subclavian artery as it travels under the clavicle and ribs.

GERBER'S TEST (LIFT-OFF TEST)

TEST POSITIONING

The subject sits or stands with the humerus internally rotated and the hand placed behind the back. The examiner stands directly behind the subject (Figure S3-34A).

ACTION

The examiner asks the subject to lift the hand off the back (Figure S3-34B).

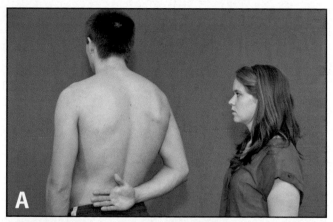

Figure S3-34A.

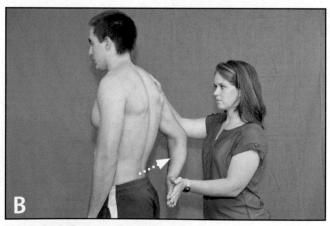

Figure S3-34B.

POSITIVE FINDING

A tear or weakness of the subscapularis is suspected if the subject cannot lift the hand off the back.

SPECIAL CONSIDERATIONS/COMMENTS

Some subjects may find this positioning uncomfortable, so it is suggested that it be used only in people with acceptable internal rotation range of motion.

EVIDENCE

	Hegedus et al (2008)	Hegedus (2012)
Study design	Systematic review	Systematic review
Conditions evaluated	Rotator cuff pathology	Rotator cuff pathology
Study number	5	11
Reliability	Not evaluated	Not evaluated
Sensitivity	17 to 92	6 to 69
Specificity	60 to 98	23 to 90

REFERENCES

Hegedus EJ. Which physical examination tests provide clinicians with the most value when examining the shoulder? Update of a systematic review with meta-analysis of individual tests. *Br J Sports Med.* 2012;46(14):964-978.

Hegedus EJ, Goode A, Campbell S, et al. Physical examination tests of the shoulder: a systematic review with meta-analysis of individual tests. *Br J Sports Med.* 2008;42(2):80-92; discussion 92.

SHOULDER

JERK TEST (POSTERIOR STRESS)

TEST POSITIONING

The subject is seated. The examiner stands behind and to the side of the subject (Figure S3-35A), with one hand stabilizing the subject's scapula and the other hand supporting the shoulder in internal rotation and 90 degrees of flexion and the elbow in position of 90 degrees of flexion.

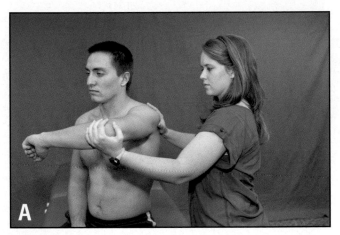

Figure S3-35A.

ACTION

The examiner passively moves the subject's arm into horizontal adduction while also placing an axial load on the humerus (Figure S3-35B).

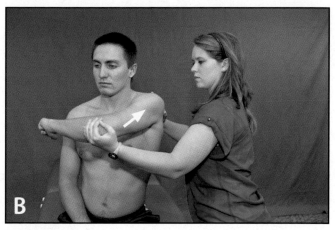

Figure S3-35B.

POSITIVE FINDING

Posterior instability is suspected if the subject experiences a painful or nonpainful clunk.

SPECIAL CONSIDERATIONS/COMMENTS

It is important to be sure the subject is relaxed so the passive motion and axial load can be applied correctly. Additionally, subjects with a positive test should also be evaluated for a posteroinferior labral tear.

EVIDENCE

	Hegedus et al (2008)
Study design	Systematic review
Conditions evaluated	Labral pathologies
Study number	2
Reliability	Not evaluated
Sensitivity	25 to 73
Specificity	80 to 98

REFERENCES

Hegedus EJ, Goode A, Campbell S, et al. Physical examination tests of the shoulder: a systematic review with meta-analysis of individual tests. *Br J Sports Med.* 2008;42(2):80-92; discussion 92.

Kim SH, Park JS, Jeong WK, Shin SK. The Kim test: a novel test for posteroinferior labral lesion of the shoulder—a comparison to the jerk test. *Am J Sports Med.* 2005;33(8):1188-1192.

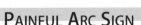

PAINFUL ARC SIGN

TEST POSITIONING

The subject and the examiner stand facing each other.

ACTION

The examiner asks the subject to actively abduct the arm (Figure S3-36).

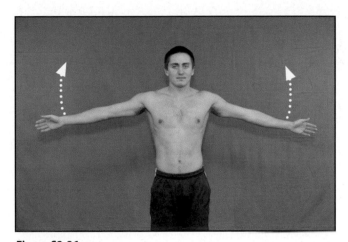

Figure S3-36.

POSITIVE FINDING

Impingement is suspected if the subject reports pain when reaching 60 to 120 degrees of arm abduction.

SPECIAL CONSIDERATIONS/COMMENTS

Although this test can be completed in a standing position, it is also possible for subjects to perform this test in a seated position. Additionally, pain experienced outside of the 60- to 120-degree range are considered a negative result for impingement.

EVIDENCE

	Hegedus et al (2008)	Hegedus (2012)
Study design	Systematic review	Meta-analysis
Conditions evaluated	Impingement syndrome	Impingement syndrome
Study number	2	4
Sample size		756
Reliability	Not evaluated	Not evaluated
Sensitivity	10 to 74	53
Specificity	47 to 88	76

REFERENCES

Hegedus EJ. Which physical examination tests provide clinicians with the most value when examining the shoulder? Update of a systematic review with meta-analysis of individual tests. *Br J Sports Med.* 2012;46(14): 964-978.

Hegedus EJ, Goode A, Campbell S, et al. Physical examination tests of the shoulder: a systematic review with meta-analysis of individual tests. *Br J Sports Med.* 2008;42(2):80-92; discussion 92.

Kessel L, Watson M. The painful arc syndrome. Clinical classification as a guide to management. *J Bone Joint Surg Br.* 1977;59(2):166-172.

Park HB, Yokota A, Gill HS, El Rassi G, McFarland EG. Diagnostic accuracy of clinical tests for the different degrees of subacromial impingement syndrome. *J Bone Joint Surg Am.* 2005;87(7):1446-1455.

Please see videos on the accompanying website at
www.healio.com/books/specialtestsvideos

Section

4

Elbow

Guide to Figures

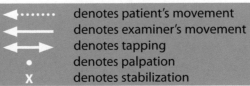

◄┈┈┈┈   denotes patient's movement

◄─────   denotes examiner's movement

◄────►   denotes tapping

•   denotes palpation

x   denotes stabilization

Konin JG, Lebsack D, Snyder Valier AR, Isear JA Jr.
Special Tests for Orthopedic Examination, Fourth Edition (pp 101-120).
© 2016 SLACK Incorporated.

RESISTIVE TENNIS ELBOW TEST (COZEN'S TEST)

TEST POSITIONING

The subject sits. The examiner stabilizes the involved elbow while palpating along the lateral epicondyle (Figure E4-1A).

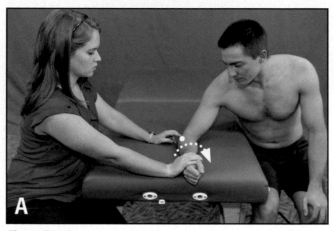

Figure E4-1A.

ACTION

With a closed fist, the subject pronates and radially deviates the forearm and extends the wrist against the examiner's resistance (Figure E4-1B).

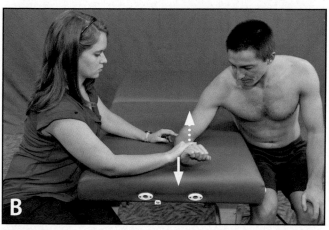

Figure E4-1B.

POSITIVE FINDING

A report of pain along the lateral epicondyle region of the humerus or objective muscle weakness as a result of complaints of discomfort may indicate lateral epicondylitis.

REFERENCES

Budoff JE, Nirschl RP. Office examination of the elbow: how provocative tests can help clinch the diagnosis. *Consultant.* 2001;41:7.

Peterson M, Butler S, Eriksson M, Svärdsudd K. A randomized controlled trial of exercise versus wait-list in chronic tennis elbow (lateral epicondylosis). *Ups J Med Sci.* 116(4):269-279.

RESISTIVE TENNIS ELBOW TEST

TEST POSITIONING

The subject sits. The examiner stabilizes the involved elbow with one hand and places the palm of the other hand on the dorsal aspect of the subject's hand just distal to the proximal interphalangeal joint of the third digit (Figure E4-2).

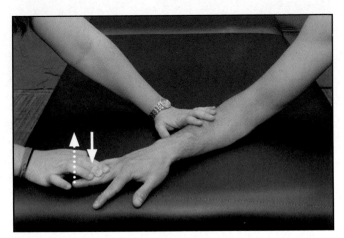

Figure E4-2.

ACTION

The subject extends the third digit against the examiner's resistance.

POSITIVE FINDING

A reporting of pain along the lateral epicondyle region of the humerus or objective muscle weakness as a result of complaints of discomfort may indicate lateral epicondylitis.

SPECIAL CONSIDERATIONS/COMMENTS

Clinicians have reported differentiating between the extensor carpi radialis longus (resistance over the second metacarpal) and the extensor carpi radialis brevis (resistance over the third metacarpal). Although this may be possible, often both may present with a positive finding and the area of local palpable tenderness is at or near the lateral epicondyle.

REFERENCE

Budoff JE, Nirschl RP. Office examination of the elbow: how provocative tests can help clinch the diagnosis. *Consultant.* 2001;41:7.

PASSIVE TENNIS ELBOW TEST

TEST POSITIONING

The subject sits with the involved elbow in full extension.

ACTION

The examiner passively pronates the forearm and flexes the subject's wrist (Figure E4-3A).

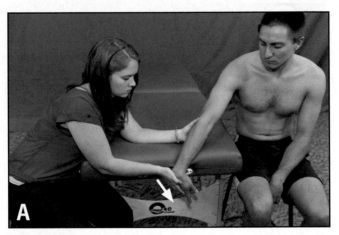

Figure E4-3A.

POSITIVE FINDING

A reporting of pain along the lateral epicondyle region of the humerus may indicate lateral epicondylitis.

SPECIAL CONSIDERATIONS/COMMENTS

The examiner may also palpate the involved lateral epicondyle region during the test to assess the tightness of the common extensor tendon origin. This test may also be performed with the elbow in flexion (Figure E4-3B).

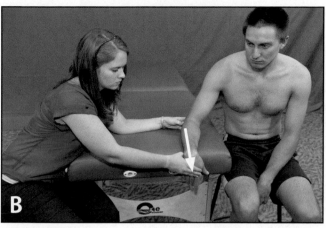

Figure E4-3B.

ELBOW

GOLFER'S ELBOW TEST

TEST POSITIONING

The subject sits or stands and makes a fist on the involved side. The examiner faces the subject and palpates along the medial epicondyle. The examiner's other hand grasps the subject's wrist (Figure E4-4A).

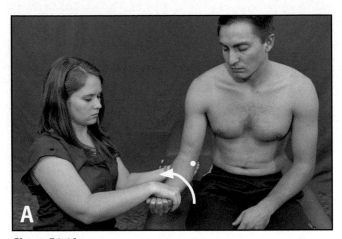

Figure E4-4A.

ACTION

The examiner passively supinates the forearm and extends the elbow and wrist (Figure E4-4B).

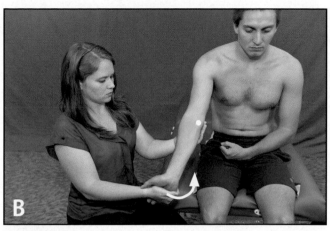

Figure E4-4B.

POSITIVE FINDING

Complaints of discomfort along the medial aspect of the elbow may be indicative of medial epicondylitis.

SPECIAL CONSIDERATIONS/COMMENTS

Pain along the medial epicondyle region of the involved elbow may also be caused by structural damage to the ulnar nerve or the ulnar collateral ligament. It is important to assess each of these structures prior to making any conclusive determinations from this test alone.

HYPEREXTENSION TEST

TEST POSITIONING

The subject sits or stands with the elbow fully extended and the forearm supinated. The examiner grasps the distal humerus at the areas of the medial and lateral epicondyles with one hand while the other hand grasps the distal forearm of the subject (Figure E4-5).

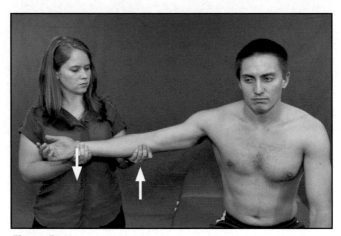

Figure E4-5.

ACTION

The examiner passively extends the elbow until no further motion is available.

POSITIVE FINDING

Elbow extension beyond 0 degrees is considered hyperextension. A positive finding of hyperextension may be attributed to a torn or stretched anterior capsule of the elbow.

SPECIAL CONSIDERATIONS/COMMENTS

Assessing this motion should always be performed bilaterally to determine the normal range of motion for the individual subject. Hyperextension findings may vary depending on the type of end-feel noted.

ELBOW

ELBOW FLEXION TEST

TEST POSITIONING

The subject may sit or stand. The examiner stands next to the subject.

ACTION

The subject is instructed to maximally flex the elbow and hold this position for 3 to 5 minutes (Figure E4-6).

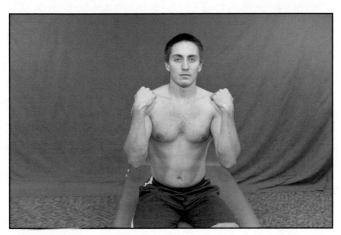

Figure E4-6.

POSITIVE FINDING

Radiating pain into the median nerve distribution in the subject's arm and/or hand (ie, lateral forearm or tip of thumb, index and middle finger, lateral half of index finger) is a positive finding. A positive test is indicative of cubital fossa syndrome.

SPECIAL CONSIDERATIONS/COMMENTS

This test may also be indicative of ulnar nerve compromise in the ulnar groove if radiating pain extends into the subject's ulnar nerve distribution (ie, the fifth digit and the medial aspect of the fourth digit).

EVIDENCE

	Ochi et al (2011)	Novak et al (1994)
Study design	Diagnostic accuracy	Diagnostic accuracy
Conditions evaluated	Cubital tunnel syndrome	Cubital tunnel syndrome
Sample size	93	65
Reliability	Not evaluated	Not evaluated
Sensitivity	36	32 to 75
Specificity	1	99

REFERENCES

Black BT, Barron OA, Townsend PF, Glickel SZ, Eaton RG. Stabilized subcutaneous ulnar nerve transposition with immediate range of motion: long-term follow-up. *J Bone Joint Surg Am.* 2000;82-A(11):1544-1551.

Cohen MS, Garfin SR. Nerve compression syndromes: finding the cause of upper-extremity symptoms. *Consultant.* 1997;37(2):241-254.

Norkus SA, Meyers MC. Ulnar neuropathy of the elbow. *Sports Med.* 1994;17(3):189-199.

Novak CB, Lee GW, Mackinnon SE, Lay L. Provocative testing for cubital tunnel syndrome. *J Hand Surg Am.* 1994;19(5):817-820.

Ochi K, Horiuchi Y, Tanabe A, Morita K, Takeda K, Ninomiya K. Comparison of shoulder internal rotation test with the elbow flexion test in the diagnosis of cubital tunnel syndrome. *J Hand Surg Am.* 2011;36(5):782-787.

ELBOW

VARUS STRESS TEST

TEST POSITIONING

The subject sits with the test elbow flexed from 20 to 30 degrees. The examiner stands with the distal hand around subject's wrist (laterally) and the proximal hand over the subject's elbow joint (medially) (Figure E4-7).

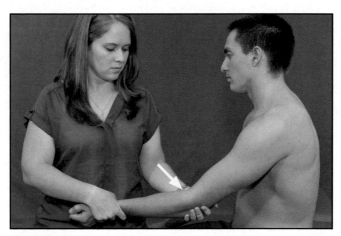

Figure E4-7.

ACTION

With the wrist stabilized, the examiner applies a varus stress to the elbow with the proximal hand.

POSITIVE FINDING

As compared to the uninvolved elbow, lateral elbow pain and/or increased varus movement with a diminished or absent endpoint is indicative of damage primarily to the radial (lateral) collateral ligament.

SPECIAL CONSIDERATIONS/COMMENTS

The examiner must avoid allowing the humerus to internally or externally rotate during this test because this will give the illusion of increased varus movement.

VALGUS STRESS TEST

TEST POSITIONING

The subject sits with the test elbow flexed from 20 to 30 degrees. The examiner stands with the distal hand around the subject's wrist (medially) and the proximal hand over the subject's elbow joint (laterally) (Figure E4-8).

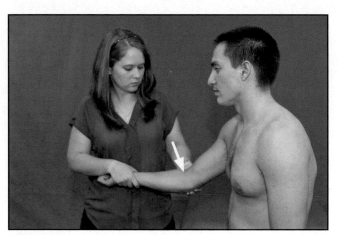

Figure E4-8.

ACTION

With the wrist stabilized, the examiner applies a valgus stress to the elbow with the proximal hand.

POSITIVE FINDING

As compared to the uninvolved elbow, medial elbow and/or increased valgus movement with a diminished or absent endpoint is indicative of damage to primarily the ulnar (medial) collateral ligament.

SPECIAL CONSIDERATIONS/COMMENTS

The examiner must avoid allowing the humerus to internally or externally rotate during this test because this will give the illusion of increased valgus movement.

EVIDENCE

	Ellenbecker and Boeckmann (1998)
Study design	Reliability
Conditions evaluated	Medial elbow laxity
Sample size	37
Reliability	ICC = .33 to .6
Sensitivity	Not evaluated
Specificity	Not evaluated

REFERENCES

Budoff JE, Nirschl RP. Office examination of the elbow: palpation and instability tests. *Consultant.* 2001;41(6):878-886.

Ellenbecker TS, Boeckmann RR. Interrater reliability of manual valgus stress testing of the elbow joint and its relation to an objective stress: radiography technique in professional baseball pitchers. *J Orthop Sports Phys Ther.* 1998;27(1):95.

Inoue G, Kuwahata Y. Surgical repair of traumatic medial disruption of the elbow in competitive athletes. *Br J Sports Med.* 1995;29(2):139-142.

O'Driscoll SW. Classification and evaluation of recurrent instability of the elbow. *Clin Orthop.* 2000;370:34-43.

Schnenck R Jr, ed. *Athletic Training and Sports Medicine.* Rosemont, IL: American Academy of Orthopedic Surgeons; 1997.

ELBOW

TINEL'S SIGN

TEST POSITIONING

The subject is seated with the elbow in slight flexion, and the examiner is standing with the distal hand grasping the subject's wrist (laterally).

ACTION

With the wrist stabilized, tap the ulnar nerve in the ulnar notch (between the olecranon process and medial epicondyle) with 1 or 2 fingers (Figure E4-9).

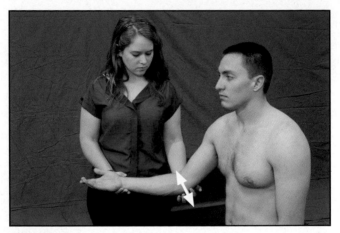

Figure E4-9.

POSITIVE FINDING

Tingling along the ulnar distribution of the forearm, hand, and fingers is indicative of ulnar nerve compromise.

Special Considerations/Comments

A positive finding can be related to traction of the ulnar nerve from a valgus force or it can be related to some type of compression of the nerve itself, as would be seen with inflammation surrounding the area. Performance of a bilateral assessment is recommended for comparison of results.

Evidence

	Beekman et al (2009)	Cheng et al (2008)
Study design	Cohort	Diagnostic accuracy
Conditions evaluated	Ulnar neuropathy at the elbow	Carpal and cubital tunnel syndrome
Sample size	192	169
Reliability	Not evaluated	Not evaluated
Sensitivity	62	32
Specificity	53	99

References

Alfonso MI, Dzwierzynski W. Tinel's sign: the realities. *Phys Med Rehabil Clin N Am.* 1998;9(4):721-736.

Beekman R, Schreuder AH, Rozeman CA, Koehler PJ, Uitdehaag BM. The diagnostic value of provocative clinical tests in ulnar neuropathy at the elbow is marginal. *J Neurol Neurosurg Psychiatry.* 2009;80(12):1369-1374.

Black BT, Barron OA, Townsend PF, Glickel SZ, Eaton RG. Stabilized subcutaneous ulnar nerve transposition with immediate range of motion. Long-term follow-up. *J Bone Joint Surg Am.* 2000;82-A(11):1544-1551.

Cheng CJ, Mackinnon-Patterson B, Beck JL, Mackinnon SE. Scratch collapse test for evaluation of carpal and cubital tunnel syndrome. *J Hand Surg Am.* 2008;33(9):1518-1524.

D'Arcy CA, McGee S. Does this patient have carpal tunnel syndrome? *JAMA.* 2000;283(23):3110-3117.

Durkan JA. A new diagnostic test for carpal tunnel syndrome. *J Bone Joint Surg Am.* 1992;73(4):535-538.

Garfinkel MS, Singhal A, Katz WA, Allan DA, Reshetar R, Schumacher HR Jr. Yoga-based intervention for carpal tunnel syndrome: a randomized trial. *JAMA.* 1998;280(18):1601-1603.

Gianni F, Mondelli M, Passero S. Provocative tests in different stages of carpal tunnel syndrome. *Clin Neurosurg.* 2001;103(3):178-183.

Kingery WS, Park KS, Wu PB, Date ES. Electromyographic motor Tinel's sign in ulnar mononeuropathies at the elbow. *Am J Phys Med Rehabil.* 1995;74(6):419-426.

Kuhlman KA, Hennessey WJ. Sensitivity and specificity of carpal tunnel syndrome signs. *Am J Phys Med Rehabil.* 1997;76(6):451-457.

Monsivais JJ, Sun Y. Tinel's sign or percussion test? Developing a better method of evoking a Tinel's sign. *J South Orthop Assoc.* 1997;6(3):186-189.

Montagna P, Liguori R. The motor Tinel's sign: a useful sign in entrapment neuropathy? *Muscle Nerve.* 2000;23(6):976-978.

Pearce JM. Tinel's sign of formication. *J Neurol Neurosurg Psychiatry.* 1996;61(1):61.

Spicher C, Kohut G, Miauton J. At which stage of sensory recovery can a tingling sign be expected? A review and proposal for standardization and grading. *J Hand Ther.* 1999;12(4):298-308.

Stolp-Smith KA, Pascoe MK, Ogburn PL Jr. Carpal tunnel syndrome in pregnancy: frequency, severity, and prognosis. *Arch Phys Med Rehabil.* 1998;79(10):1285-1287.

ELBOW

Pinch Grip Test

Test Positioning

The subject may sit or stand. The examiner stands next to the subject.

Action

The subject is instructed to pinch the tips of the thumb and index finger together (Figure E4-10).

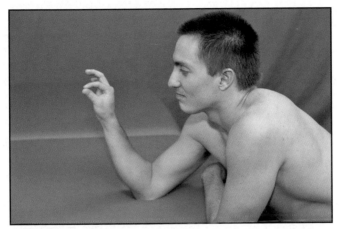

Figure E4-10.

Positive Finding

The inability to touch the pads of the thumb and index finger together demonstrates a positive finding. Touching the pads of the thumb and index finger indicates function of the anterior interosseous nerve between the 2 heads of the pronator muscle.

Special Considerations/Comments

The anterior interosseous nerve is a branch of the median nerve (C7 to C8, T1) that innervates the pronator quadratus, flexor pollicis longus, and the first and second components of the flexor digitorum profundus.

REFERENCE

Thurston A, Lam N. Results of open carpal tunnel release: a comprehensive, retrospective study of 188 hands. *Aust N Z Surg*. 1997;67(5):283-288.

ELBOW

Please see videos on the accompanying website at
www.healio.com/books/specialtestsvideos

Section

5

Wrist and Hand

Guide to Figures

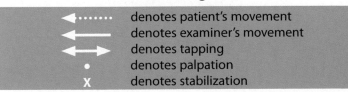

denotes patient's movement
denotes examiner's movement
denotes tapping
denotes palpation
denotes stabilization

Konin JG, Lebsack D, Snyder Valier AR, Isear JA Jr.
Special Tests for Orthopedic Examination, Fourth Edition (pp 121-155).
© 2016 SLACK Incorporated.

TAP OR PERCUSSION TEST

TEST POSITIONING

The subject may sit or stand with the affected finger extended. The examiner stands in front of the subject.

ACTION

The examiner applies a firm tap to the end of the finger being tested (Figure WH5-1A). As an alternative method to tapping, the examiner may use a percussion hammer (Figure WH5-1B).

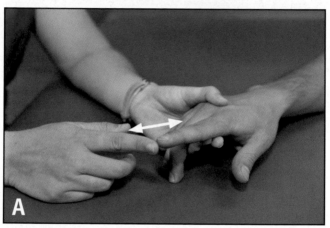

Figure WH5-1A.

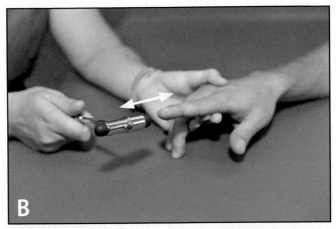

Figure WH5-1B.

POSITIVE FINDING

Pain at the site of injury indicates a fracture. The vibration of tapping along the long axis of the bone will exaggerate pain at the fracture site.

SPECIAL CONSIDERATIONS/COMMENTS

This test should not be performed if there is an obvious deformity.

COMPRESSION TEST

TEST POSITIONING

The subject may sit or stand with the affected finger extended. The examiner stands in front of the subject.

ACTION

The examiner holds the distal phalanx and applies compression along the long axis of the bone of the finger being tested (Figure WH5-2).

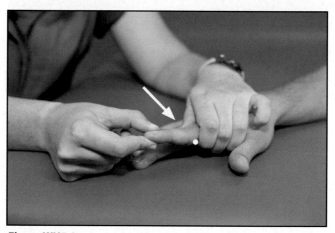

Figure WH5-2.

POSITIVE FINDING

Pain at the site of injury indicates a fracture.

SPECIAL CONSIDERATIONS/COMMENTS

This test should not be performed if there is an obvious deformity.

REFERENCE

Tetro AM, Evanoff BA, Hollstien SB, Gelberman RH. A new provocative test for carpal tunnel syndrome. Assessment of wrist flexion and nerve compression. *J Bone Joint Surg Br.* 1998;80(3):493-498.

WRIST AND HAND

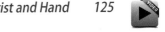

LONG FINGER FLEXION TEST

TEST POSITIONING

The subject may sit or stand.

ACTION

1. The examiner stands in front of the subject and holds the subject's fingers in extension, except for the finger being tested.
2. The examiner isolates the distal interphalangeal joint by stabilizing the metacarpophalangeal joint, proximal interphalangeal joints, and middle phalanx of the finger being tested.
3. The subject is instructed to flex the finger being tested at the distal interphalangeal joint (Figure WH5-3A).

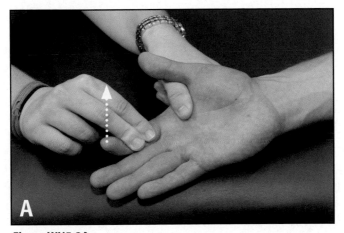

Figure WH5-3A.

4. Next, the examiner isolates the proximal interphalangeal joint by stabilizing the metacarpophalangeal joint and the proximal phalanx. The subject is then instructed to flex the proximal interphalangeal joint (Figure WH5-3B).

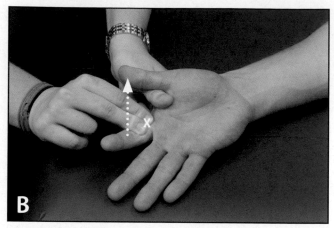

Figure WH5-3B. Note: Stabilize at the proximal joint.

POSITIVE FINDING

If the subject is unable to flex the proximal interphalangeal joint, then both the flexor digitorum profundus and the flexor digitorum superficialis muscles' tendon and/or nerve are compromised. If the subject is able to flex the proximal interphalangeal joint but is unable to flex the distal interphalangeal joint, then only the flexor digitorum muscle's tendon and/or nerve are compromised.

SPECIAL CONSIDERATIONS/COMMENTS

The examiner should always perform passive flexion to both the proximal and distal interphalangeal joints to be sure that an inability to flex these joints is not related to soft tissue tightness or joint restrictions. This test should not be repeated multiple times if a tendon rupture is suspected.

FINKELSTEIN TEST

TEST POSITIONING

The subject sits or stands and forms a fist around the thumb. The examiner stands with the proximal hand grasping the subject's forearm and the distal hand grasping the subject's fist.

ACTION

While stabilizing the subject's forearm with the proximal hand, ulnarly deviate the subject's wrist with the distal hand (Figure WH5-4A).

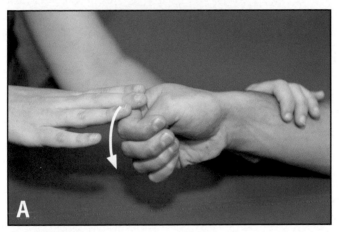

Figure WH5-4A.

POSITIVE FINDING

Pain over the abductor pollicis longus and extensor pollicis brevis tendons distally is indicative of tenosynovitis in these tendons (de Quervain's disease).

SPECIAL CONSIDERATIONS/COMMENTS

This test may create pain in uninvolved tissues. The examiner may also find that simple passive ulnar deviation may be slightly uncomfortable for even those without pathology. If de Quervain's disease is suspected, but pain is not found with ulnar deviation, then the examiner can have the subject radially deviate against resistance in an attempt to reproduce contractile-associated pain (Figure WH5-4B).

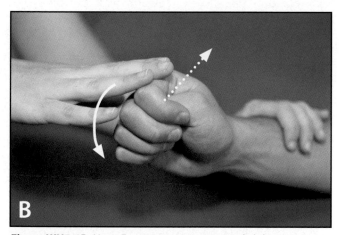

Figure WH5-4B. Note: Examiner resists active radial deviation.

REFERENCES

Dawson C, Mudgal CS. Staged description of the Finkelstein test. *J Hand Surg Am.* 2010;35(9):1513-1515.

Elliot BG. Finkelstein's test: a descriptive error that can produce a false positive. *J Hand Surg Br.* 1992;17(4):481-482.

Murtagh J. De Quervain's tenosynovitis and Finkelstein's test. *Aust Fam Physician.* 1989;18(12):1552.

WRIST AND HAND

PHALEN TEST

TEST POSITIONING

The subject sits or stands with the dorsal aspect of both hands in full contact so that both wrists are maximally flexed (Figure WH5-5).

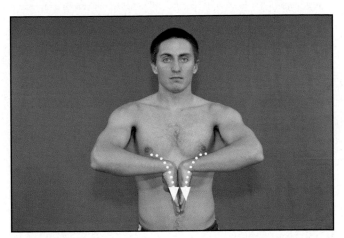

Figure WH5-5.

ACTION

A steady compressive force is applied through the subject's forearms so the subject's wrists are maximally flexed for 1 minute.

POSITIVE FINDING

Numbness and tingling in the median nerve distribution of the fingers (ie, thumb, index finger, middle finger, and lateral aspect of the ring finger) are indicative of carpal tunnel syndrome secondary to median nerve compression.

SPECIAL CONSIDERATIONS/COMMENTS

Pain in the wrist area, without complaints of radiating pain distally toward the hand and fingers, may be indicative of carpal bone pathology.

EVIDENCE

	Wainner et al (2005)	El Miedany et al (2008)	Ma and Kim (2012)
Study design	Diagnostic accuracy	Diagnostic accuracy	Diagnostic accuracy
Conditions evaluated	Cervical radiculopathy or carpal tunnel syndrome	Carpal tunnel syndrome and tenosynovitis	Carpal tunnel syndrome
Sample size	82	232	38
Reliability	Kappa = .79	Not evaluated	Not evaluated
Sensitivity	77	Carpal tunnel: 47 Tenosynovitis: 92	84
Specificity	40	Carpal tunnel: 17 Tenosynovitis: 87	87

REFERENCES

Burke DT, Burke MA, Bell R, Stewart GW, Mehdi RS, Kim HJ. Subjective swelling: a new sign for carpal tunnel syndrome. *Am J Phys Med Rehabil.* 1999;78(6):504-508.

El Miedany Y, Ashour S, Youssef S, Mehanna A, Meky FA. Clinical diagnosis of carpal tunnel syndrome: old tests—new concepts. *Joint Bone Spine.* 2008;75(4):451-457.

Ghavanini MR, Haghighat M. Carpal tunnel syndrome: reappraisal of five clinical tests. *Electromyogr Clin Neurophysiol.* 1998;38(7):437-441.

Keniston RC, Nathan PA, Leklem JE, Lockwood RS. Vitamin B6, vitamin C, and carpal tunnel syndrome: a cross-sectional study of 441 adults. *J Occup Environ Med.* 1997;39(10):949-959.

Ma H, Kim I. The diagnostic assessment of hand elevation test in carpal tunnel syndrome. *J Korean Neurosurg Soc.* 2012;52(5):472-475.

WRIST AND HAND

Mondelli M, Passero S, Giannini F. Provocative tests in different stages of carpal tunnel syndrome. *Clin Neurol Neurosurg*. 2001;103(3):178-183.

Oporto LM, Pérez AA, Navajas RF, Puerta AG. Diagnostic value of symptoms and clinical exploration in carpal tunnel syndrome [article in Spanish]. *Rehabilitación*. 1997;31(1):23-27.

Padua L, Padua R, Aprile I, Pasqualetti P, Tonali P; for the Italian CTS Study Group. Multiperspective follow-up of untreated carpal tunnel syndrome: a multicenter study. *Neurology*. 2001;56(11):1459-1466.

Rempel D, Tittiranonda P, Burastero S, Hudes M, So Y. Effect of keyboard keyswitch design on hand pain. *J Occup Environ Med*. 1999;41(2):111-119.

Seiler JG. Carpal tunnel syndrome: update on diagnostic testing and treatment options. *Consultant*. 1997;37(5):1233.

Szabo RM, Slater RR Jr, Farver TB, Stanton DB, Sharman WK. The value of diagnostic testing in carpal tunnel syndrome. *J Hand Surg*. 1999;24(4):704-714.

Tetro AM, Evanoff BA, Hollstien SB, Gelberman RH. A new, provocative test for carpal tunnel syndrome: assessment of wrist flexion and nerve compression. *J Bone Joint Surgery Br*. 1998;80 (3):493-498.

Valdes K, LaStayo P. The value of provocative tests for the wrist and elbow: a literature review. *J Hand Ther*. 2013;26(1):32-42; quiz 43.

Wainner RS, Fritz JM, Irrgang JJ, Delitto A, Allison S, Boninger ML. Development of a clinical prediction rule for the diagnosis of carpal tunnel syndrome. *Arch Phys Med Rehabil*. 2005;86(4):609-618.

WRIST AND HAND

REVERSE PHALEN TEST

TEST POSITIONING

The subject stands or sits with the palmer aspect of both hands in full contact so both wrists are maximally extended.

ACTION

A steady compressive force is applied through the subject's forearms so that the subject's wrists are maximally extended for 1 minute (Figure WH5-6).

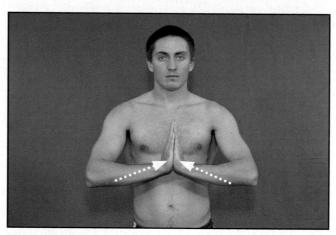

Figure WH5-6.

POSITIVE FINDING

Numbness and tingling in the median nerve distribution of the fingers (ie, thumb, index finger, middle finger, and lateral aspect of the ring finger) are indicative of carpal tunnel syndrome secondary to median nerve compression.

SPECIAL CONSIDERATIONS/COMMENTS

Pain in the wrist area without complaints of radiating pain distally toward the hand and fingers may be indicative of carpal bone pathology.

WRIST AND HAND

Evidence

	El Miedany et al (2008)
Study design	Diagnostic accuracy
Conditions evaluated	Carpal tunnel syndrome and tenosynovitis
Sample size	232
Reliability	Not evaluated
Sensitivity	Carpal tunnel: 42 Tenosynovitis: 75
Specificity	Carpal tunnel: 35 Tenosynovitis: 85

References

El Miedany Y, Ashour S, Youssef S, Mehanna A, Meky FA. Clinical diagnosis of carpal tunnel syndrome: old tests—new concepts. *Joint Bone Spine*. 2008;75(4):451-457.

Ghavanini MR, Haghighat M. Carpal tunnel syndrome: reappraisal of five clinical tests. *Electromyogr Clin Neurophysiol*. 1998;38(7):437-441.

Kanaan N, Sawaya RA. Carpal tunnel syndrome: modern diagnostic and management techniques. *Br J Gen Pract*. 2001;51(465):311-314.

TINEL'S SIGN

TEST POSITIONING

The subject sits next to a flat surface.

ACTION

The examiner taps the volar aspect of the subject's wrist over the area of the carpal tunnel (Figure WH5-7).

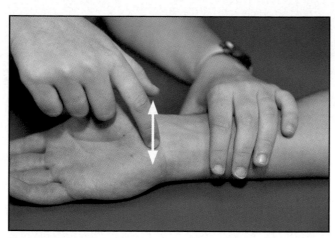

Figure WH5-7.

POSITIVE FINDING

Complaints of tingling, paresthesia, or pain by the subject in the area of the thumb, index finger, middle finger, and radial one-half of the ring finger signal a positive test. This may be indicative of a compression of the median nerve in the carpal tunnel or carpal tunnel syndrome.

SPECIAL CONSIDERATIONS/COMMENTS

A positive Tinel's sign at the wrist may appear if the median nerve is disrupted at any point of its path. Therefore, a positive finding should warrant the examiner to assess the integrity of the median nerve at the elbow, shoulder, and neck to rule out other pathologies.

EVIDENCE

	Ma and Kim (2012)	Cheng et al (2008)	Wainner et al (2005)
Study design	Diagnostic accuracy	Diagnostic accuracy	Diagnostic accuracy
Conditions evaluated	Carpal tunnel syndrome	Carpal and cubital tunnel syndrome	Carpal tunnel syndrome and cervical radiculopathy
Sample size	38	169	82
Reliability	Not evaluated	Not evaluated	Kappa = .35 to .47
Sensitivity	82	32	41 to 48
Specificity	89	99	58 to 67

REFERENCES

Alfonso MI, Dzwierzynski W. Hoffman-Tinel's sign: the realities. *Phys Med Rehabil Clin N Am.* 1998;9(4):721-736. v.

Bailie DS, Kelikian AS. Tarsal tunnel syndrome: diagnosis, surgical technique, and functional outcome. *Foot Ankle Int.* 1998;19(2):65-72.

Campbell LS. Commentary on carpal-tunnel syndrome [original article appears in *Am J Nurs.* 1993;93(4):64]. *ENA's Nursing Scan in Emergency Care.* 1993;3(5):5.

Cheng CJ, Mackinnon-Patterson B, Beck JL, Mackinnon SE. Scratch collapse test for evaluation of carpal and cubital tunnel syndrome. *J Hand Surg Am.* 2008;33(9):1518-1524.

D'Arcy CA, McGee S. Does this patient have carpal tunnel syndrome? *JAMA.* 2000;283(23):3110-3117.

El Miedany Y, Ashour S, Youssef S, Mehanna A, Meky FA. Clinical diagnosis of carpal tunnel syndrome: old tests-new concepts. *Joint Bone Spine.* 2008;75(4):451-457.

Ghavanini MR, Haghighat M. Carpal tunnel syndrome: reappraisal of five clinical tests. *Electromyogr Clin Neurophysiol.* 1998;38(7):437-441.

Goloborod'ko SA. Provocative test for carpal tunnel syndrome. *J Hand Ther.* 2004;17(3):344-348.

Katz JN, Losina E, Amick BC III, Fossel AH, Bessette L, Keller RB. Predictors of outcomes of carpal tunnel release. *Arthritis Rheum.* 2001;44(5):1184-1193.

Kuhlman KA, Hennessey WJ. Sensitivity and specificity of carpal tunnel syndrome signs. *Am J Phys Med Rehabil.* 1997;76(6):451-457.

LeBlond RF. Clinical diagnosis of carpal tunnel syndrome. *JAMA.* 2000;284(15):1924-1925.

Lord RW Jr. How accurate are the history and physical examination in diagnosing carpal tunnel syndrome? *J Fam Prac.* 2000;49(9):782-783.

Ma H, Kim I. The diagnostic assessment of hand elevation test in carpal tunnel syndrome. *J Korean Neurosurg Soc.* 2012;52(5):472-475.

Moldaver J. Tinel's sign. Its characteristics and significance. *J Bone Joint Surg Am.* 1978;60(3):412-414.

Nishikawa T, Kurosaka M, Mitani M, Matsubara N, Harada T, Mizuno K. Ulnar bursa distention following volar subluxation of the distal radioulnar joint after distal radial fracture: a rare cause of carpal tunnel syndrome. *J Orthop Trauma.* 2001;15(6):450-452.

Seiler JG. Carpal tunnel syndrome: update on diagnostic testing and treatment options. *Consultant.* 1997;37(5):1233.

Shergill G, Bonney G, Munshi P, Birch R. The radial and posterior interosseous nerves. Results of 260 repairs. *J Bone Joint Surg Br.* 2001;83(5):646-649.

Wainner RS, Fritz JM, Irrgang JJ, Delitto A, Allison S, Boninger ML. Development of a clinical prediction rule for the diagnosis of carpal tunnel syndrome. *Arch Phys Med Rehabil.* 2005;86(4):609-618.

WRIST
AND HAND

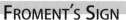

FROMENT'S SIGN

TEST POSITIONING

The subject may sit or stand. The examiner sits next to the subject.

ACTION

The subject is instructed to hold a piece of paper between the thumb and index finger. The examiner then tries to pull the paper out (Figure WH5-8).

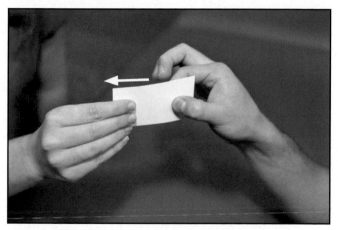

Figure WH5-8.

POSITIVE FINDING

Flexion of the distal interphalangeal joint of the subject's thumb is indicative of adductor pollicis muscle paralysis due to ulnar nerve damage.

SPECIAL CONSIDERATIONS/COMMENTS

Simultaneous hyperextension of the metacarpophalangeal joint of the thumb is indicative of ulnar nerve compromise. This is known as Jeanne's Sign.

REFERENCES

Drury W, Stern PJ. Froment's paper sign and Jeanne's sign—unusual etiology. *J Hand Surg Am*. 1982;7(4):404-406.

Goldman SB, Brininger TL, Schrader JW, Curtis R, Koceja DM. Analysis of clinical motor testing for adult patients with diagnosed ulnar neuropathy at the elbow. *Arch Phys Med Rehabil*. 2009;90(11):1846-1852.

Loréa P, Schuind F. False aneurysm appearing as delayed ulnar nerve palsy after "minor" penetrating trauma in the forearm. *J Trauma*. 2001;51(1):144-145.

Richardson C, Fabre G. Froment's sign. *J Audiov Media Med*. 2003;26(1):34.

WRIST
AND HAND

WRINKLE TEST

TEST POSITIONING

The subject sits near a flat surface.

ACTION

The subject's fingers are placed in warm water for approximately 10 minutes (Figure WH5-9). On removal, the examiner assesses the skin around the pulp area for any wrinkling.

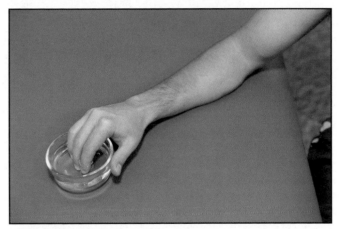

Figure WH5-9.

POSITIVE FINDING

A positive test is seen when the involved finger shows no signs of wrinkling, indicating denervated tissue.

SPECIAL CONSIDERATIONS

This test can be used as an assessment tool for documenting peripheral nerve regeneration by way of pulp-area wrinkling. Furthermore, submersion of the fourth digit may allow for one to distinguish between median and ulnar nerve pathology.

REFERENCES

Falanga V. The "wrinkle test": clinical use for detecting early epidermal resurfacing. *J Dermatol Surg Oncol.* 1993;19(2):172-173.

Vasudevan TM, van Rij AM, Nukada H, Taylor PK. Skin wrinkling for the assessment of sympathetic function in the limbs. *Aust N Z J Surg.* 2000;70(1):57-59.

DIGITAL ALLEN'S TEST

TEST POSITIONING

Both the subject and examiner may sit or stand.

ACTION

The subject is instructed to make a fist several times in succession to "pump" the blood out of the hand and fingers. The subject is then instructed to maintain a fist while the examiner compresses the radial artery and the ulnar artery (Figure WH5-10A). As the subject relaxes the hand (Figure WH5-10B), the examiner releases pressure from one artery at a time and observes the color of the hand and fingers (Figure WH5-10C).

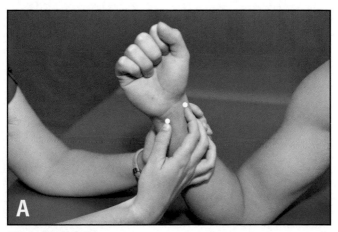

Figure WH5-10A.

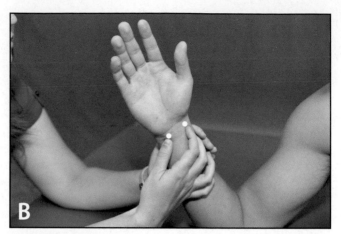

Figure WH5-10B.

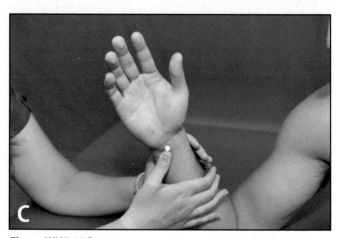

Figure WH5-10C.

Positive Finding

A delay in or absence of flushing of the radial or ulnar half of the hand and fingers is indicative of partial or complete occlusion of the radial or ulnar arteries, respectively.

Special Considerations/Comments

This test should always be performed and compared bilaterally. If a positive finding is present bilaterally, the examiner should consider brachial artery involvement.

Evidence

	Levinsohn et al (1991)
Study design	Diagnostic accuracy
Conditions evaluated	Artery occlusion
Sample size	40
Reliability	Not evaluated
Sensitivity	100
Specificity	80

References

Ashbell TS, Kutz JE, Kleinert HE. The digital Allen test. *Plast Reconstr Surg.* 1967;39(3):311-312.

Fuhrman TM, Reilley TE, Pippin WD. Comparison of digital blood pressure, plethysmography, and the modified Allen's test as means of evaluating the collateral circulation to the hand. *Anaesthesia.* 1992;47(11):959-961.

Gelberman RH, Blasingame JP. The timed Allen's test. *J Trauma.* 1981;21(6):477-479.

Lanni HA, Smith SG. Allen's test: fact or myth? *Respir Care.* 2001;46(3):274.

Levinsohn DG, Gordon L, Sessler DI. The Allen's test: analysis of four methods. *J Hand Surg Am.* 1991;16(2):279-282.

McConnell EA. Clinical do's and don'ts. Performing Allen's test....whether ulnar and radial arteries are patent. *Nursing.* 1997;27(11):26.

Pelmear PL, Kusiak R. Clinical assessment of hand-arm vibration syndrome. *Nagoya J Med Sci.* 1994;57(Suppl):27-41.

Pistorius MA, Planchon B. Diagnostic importance of digital topographic assessment of Raynaud's phenomenon. A prospective study of a population of 522 patients [article in French]. *J Mal Vasc.* 1995;20(1):14-20.

Scavenius M, Fauner M, Walther-Larsen S, Buchwald C, Nielsen SL. A quantitative Allen's test. *Hand.* 1981;13(3):318-320.

Stead SW, Stirt JA. Assessment of digital blood flow and palmar collateral circulation. Allen's test vs. photoplethysmography. *Int J Clin Monit Comput.* 1985;2(1):29-34.

Sugawara M, Ogino T, Minami A, Ishii S. Digital ischemia in baseball players. *Am J Sports Med.* 1986;14(4):329-334.

Thompson CE, Stroud SD. Allen's test: a tool for diagnosing ulnar artery trauma. *Nurse Pract.* 1984;9(12):13,16-17.

Wendt JR. Digital Allen's test as an adjunct in diagnosis of possible digital nerve lacerations. *Plast Reconstr Surg.* 1991;88(4):739-740.

WRIST AND HAND

BUNNEL LITTLER TEST

TEST POSITIONING

The subject sits with the metacarpophalangeal joint of the involved digit in slight extension.

ACTION

The examiner passively flexes the proximal interphalangeal joint of the same ray and assesses the amount of proximal interphalangeal joint flexion (Figure WH5-11A). The examiner then passively flexes the metacarpophalangeal joint slightly and again assesses the amount of flexion at the proximal interphalangeal joint (Figure WH5-11B).

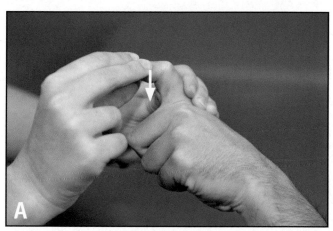

Figure WH5-11A. Note: Metacarpophalangeal joint stabilized in extension.

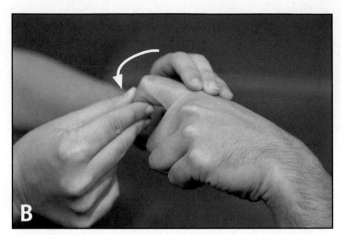

Figure WH5-11B.

POSITIVE FINDING

A positive finding is revealed if the proximal interphalangeal joint does not flex while the metacarpophalangeal joint is in an extended position. If the proximal interphalangeal joint does fully flex once the metacarpophalangeal joint is slightly flexed, intrinsic muscle tightness can be assumed. By contrast, if flexion of the proximal interphalangeal joint remains limited once the metacarpophalangeal joint is slightly flexed, capsular tightness can be assumed.

SPECIAL CONSIDERATIONS/COMMENTS

Care should be taken by the examiner to retain extension and then flexion of the metacarpophalangeal joint while also testing in each position to assess true proximal interphalangeal joint motion.

MURPHY'S SIGN

TEST POSITIONING

The subject may sit or stand. The examiner stands in front of the subject.

ACTION

The subject is instructed to make a fist. The examiner notes the position of the third metacarpal (Figure WH5-12).

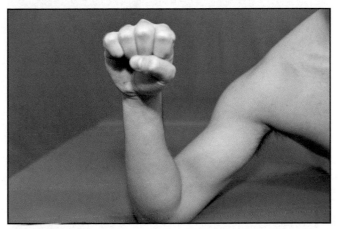

Figure WH5-12.

POSITIVE FINDING

If the subject's third metacarpal is level with the second and fourth metacarpals, a dislocated lunate is indicated.

SPECIAL CONSIDERATIONS/COMMENTS

With normal anatomical alignment, the position of the lunate makes the third metacarpal appear longer than the others when a fist is made. Thus, altering the position of the lunate in an anterior or posterior direction will allow for the third metacarpal to slide more proximally.

WRIST AND HAND

WATSON TEST

TEST POSITIONING

The subject sits. The examiner uses one hand to stabilize the distal forearm at the distal radial ulnar joint while grasping the scaphoid bone of the subject with the other hand (Figure WH5-13A).

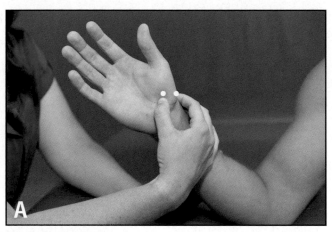

Figure WH5-13A.

ACTION

The examiner mobilizes the scaphoid bone anteriorly and posteriorly while ulnarly and radially deviating the subject's wrist (Figure WH5-13B).

WRIST
AND HAND

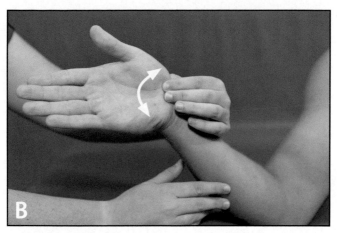

Figure WH5-13B. Note: Scaphoid is mobilized anterior/posterior while the wrist is deviated.

POSITIVE FINDING

Positive findings include a palpable subluxation and reduction of the scaphoid, and may be felt if an underlying carpal ligament tear is present.

SPECIAL CONSIDERATIONS/COMMENTS

This test is easier to perform when the examiner grasps the scaphoid on the volar aspect with the thumb. The Watson Test may also be referred to as the Scaphoid Shift Test.

EVIDENCE

	LaStayo and Howell (1995)
Study design	Diagnostic accuracy
Conditions evaluated	Wrist pain
Sample size	50
Reliability	Not evaluated
Sensitivity	69
Specificity	66

REFERENCES

Bickert B, Sauerbier M, Germann G. Clinical examination of the injured wrist [article in German]. *Zentralbl Chir.* 1997;122(11):1010-1015.

Hwang JJ, Goldfarb CA, Gelberman RH, Boyer MI. The effect of dorsal carpal ganglion excision on the scaphoid shift test. *J Hand Surg Br.* 1999;24(1):106-108.

Lane LB. The scaphoid shift test. *J Hand Surg.* 1993;18(2):366-368.

LaStayo P, Howell J. Clinical provocative tests used in evaluating wrist pain: a descriptive study. *J Hand Ther.* 1995;8(1):10-17.

Prosser R, Harvey L, LaStayo P, Hargreaves I, Scougall P, Herbert RD. Provocative wrist tests and MRI are of limited diagnostic value for suspected wrist ligament injuries: a cross-sectional study. *J Physiother.* 2011;57(4):247-253.

Sauerbier M, Tränkle M, Erdmann D, Menke H, Germann G. Functional outcome with scaphotrapeziotrapezoid arthrodesis in the treatment of Kienböck's disease stage III. *Ann Plast Surg.* 2000;44(6):618-625.

Tiel-van Buul MM, Bos KE, Dijkstra PF, van Beek EJ, Broekhuizen AH. Carpal instability, the missed diagnosis in patients with clinically suspected scaphoid fracture. *Injury.* 1993;24(4):257-262.

Valdes K, LaStayo P. The value of provocative tests for the wrist and elbow: a literature review. *J Hand Ther.* 2013;26(1):32-42; quiz 43.

Wolfe SW, Gupta A, Crisco JJ III. Kinematics of the scaphoid shift test. *J Hand Surg Am.* 1997;22(5):801-806.

WRIST AND HAND

VALGUS STRESS TEST

TEST POSITIONING

The examiner maintains stabilization of the proximal bone between the thumb and forefinger and grasps the distal bone (usually the bones comprising a hinge joint).

ACTION

The examiner provides a valgus force to the joint, creating a fulcrum while attempting to "gap the joint" (Figure WH5-14A).

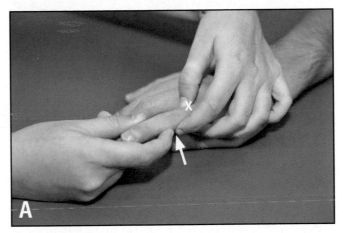

Figure WH5-14A.

POSITIVE FINDING

Any excessive gapping that is noted when compared to the uninvolved side may indicate a collateral ligament tear.

SPECIAL CONSIDERATIONS/COMMENTS

The examiner should perform this test with extreme care so no further damage is created with the valgus stress that is applied. This test can also be performed at the metacarpophalangeal joint of the thumb, where excessive joint movement would indicate an ulnar collateral ligament tear, commonly referred to as "skier's thumb" (Figure WH5-14B).

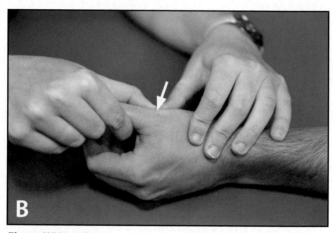

Figure WH5-14B.

VARUS STRESS TEST

TEST POSITIONING

The examiner maintains stabilization of the proximal bone between the thumb and forefinger and grasps the distal bone (usually bones comprising a hinge joint).

ACTION

The examiner provides a varus force to the joint, creating a fulcrum while attempting to "gap the joint" (Figure WH5-15).

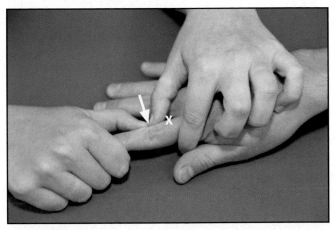

Figure WH5-15.

POSITIVE FINDING

Any excessive gapping that is noted when compared to the uninvolved side may indicate a collateral ligament tear.

SPECIAL CONSIDERATIONS/COMMENTS

The examiner should perform this test with extreme care so no further damage is created with the varus stress that is applied.

WRIST
AND HAND

BALLOTTEMENT TEST

TEST POSITIONING

The subject stands or sits. The examiner uses his or her thumb and index finger to stabilize the lunate bone of the subject's involved hand.

ACTION

While stabilizing the lunate bone, the examiner uses his or her other hand to gently move the pisotriquetral complex up and down against the lunate bone (Figure WH5-16).

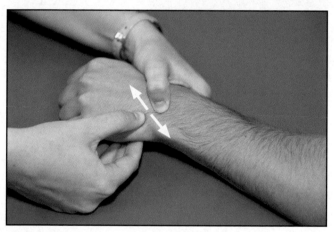

Figure WH5-16.

POSITIVE FINDING

A positive test is indicated when the subject feels pain, crepitus is produced, or excessive joint laxity is observed. Positive findings suggest lunotriquetral dissociation or ligament damage or laxity.

SPECIAL CONSIDERATIONS/COMMENTS

The area may be point tender so the testing motion should start gradually.

EVIDENCE

	LaStayo and Howell (1995)
Study design	Diagnostic accuracy
Conditions evaluated	Wrist pain
Sample size	50
Reliability	Not evaluated
Sensitivity	64
Specificity	44

REFERENCES

LaStayo P, Howell J. Clinical provocative tests used in evaluating wrist pain: a descriptive study. *J Hand Ther.* 1995;8(1):10-17.

Prosser R, Harvey L, LaStayo P, Hargreaves I, Scougall P, Herbert RD. Provocative wrist tests and MRI are of limited diagnostic value for suspected wrist ligament injuries: a cross-sectional study. *J Physiother.* 2011;57(4):247-253.

Valdes K, LaStayo P. The value of provocative tests for the wrist and elbow: a literature review. *J Hand Ther.* 2013;26(1):32-42; quiz 43.

WRIST AND HAND

Please see videos on the accompanying website at
www.healio.com/books/specialtestsvideos

Section

6

Thoracic Spine

Guide to Figures

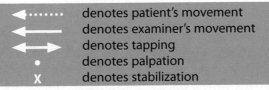

◄········ denotes patient's movement
◄──── denotes examiner's movement
◄───► denotes tapping
• denotes palpation
x denotes stabilization

Konin JG, Lebsack D, Snyder Valier AR, Isear JA Jr.
Special Tests for Orthopedic Examination, Fourth Edition (pp 157-163).
© 2016 SLACK Incorporated.

KERNIG/BRUDZINSKI SIGNS

TEST POSITIONING

The subject lies supine with his or her hands cupped behind the head. The examiner stands next to the subject.

ACTION

The subject is instructed to flex the cervical spine by lifting the head. Each hip is unilaterally flexed to no more than 90 degrees by the subject. The subject then flexes the knee to no more than 90 degrees. The opposite leg remains on the examining table (Figure TS6-1).

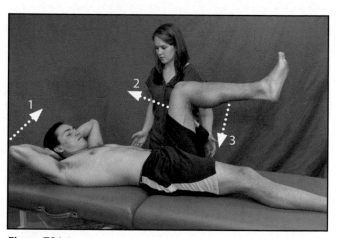

Figure TS6-1.

POSITIVE FINDING

The test is confirmed by increased pain (that is either localized or radiates into the lower extremity) with neck and hip flexion. The pain is relieved when the knee is flexed. The pain is indicative of meningeal irritation, nerve root impingement, or dural irritation that is exaggerated by elongating the spinal cord.

SPECIAL CONSIDERATIONS/COMMENTS

The considerations are similar to the straight leg raise test except the neck is flexed and the hip is actively flexed. The neck flexion component of this test was developed by Kernig, and the hip flexion component was developed by Brudzinski.

EVIDENCE

	Thomas et al (2002)	Bilavsky et al (2013)
Study design	Diagnostic accuracy	Diagnostic accuracy
Conditions evaluated	Meningitis	Meningitis
Sample size	297	86
Reliability	Not evaluated	Not evaluated
Sensitivity	Kernig sign = 5 Brudzinski sign = 5	Kernig sign = 51 Brudzinski sign = 53
Specificity	Kernig sign = 95 Brudzinski sign = 95	Kernig sign = 95 Brudzinski sign = 78

REFERENCES

Bilavsky E, Leibovitz E, Elkon-Tamir E, Fruchtman Y, Ifergan G, Greenberg D. The diagnostic accuracy of the 'classic meningeal signs' in children with suspected bacterial meningitis. *Eur J Emerg Med*. 2013;20(5):361-363.

Brody IA, Wilkins RH. The signs of Kernig and Brudzinski. *Arch Neurol*. 1969;21(2):215-218.

Mehndiratta MM, Nayak R, Garg H, Kumar M, Pandey S. Appraisal of Kernig's and Brudzinski's sign in meningitis. *Ann Indian Acad Neurol*. 2013;15(4):287-288.

Pullen RL Jr. Assessing for signs of meningitis. *Nursing*. 2004;34(5): 18.

Thomas KE, Hasbun R, Jekel J, Quagliarello VJ. The diagnostic accuracy of Kernig's sign, Brudzinski's sign, and nuchal rigidity in adults with suspected meningitis. *Clin Infect Dis*. 2002;35(1):46-52.

THORACIC SPINE

Verghese A, Gallemore G. Kernig's and Brudzinski's signs revisited. *Rev Infect Dis*. 1987;9(6):1187-1192.

Ward MA, Greenwood TM, Kumar DR, Mazza JJ, Yale SH. Josef Brudzinski and Vladimir Mikhailovich Kernig: signs for diagnosing meningitis. *Clin Med Res*. 2010;8(1):13-17.

Wartenberg R. Lasègue sign and Kernig sign; historical notes. *AMA Arch Neurol Psychiatry*. 1951;66(1):58-60.

Wartenberg R. The signs of Brudzinski and of Kernig. *J Pediatr*. 1950;37(4):679-684.

LATERAL AND ANTERIOR/POSTERIOR RIB COMPRESSION TESTS

TEST POSITIONING

1. The subject lies supine. The examiner stands next to the subject and places a hand on either side of the affected rib(s) (Figure TS6-2A).

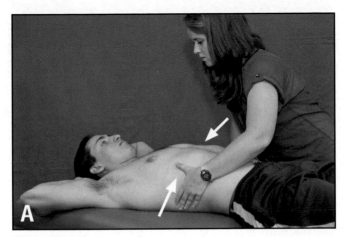

Figure TS6-2A.

2. The subject lies supine. The examiner stands next to the subject and places one hand over the affected rib(s) and the other hand posterior to the rib cage (Figure TS6-2B).

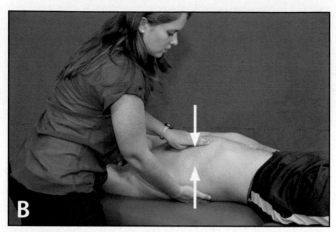

Figure TS6-2B.

ACTION

1. The examiner compresses the lateral aspect of the rib cage bilaterally and then quickly releases.
2. The examiner compresses the rib cage anterior to posterior and quickly releases.

POSITIVE FINDING

Pain with compression or release of pressure indicates the possibility of a rib fracture, rib contusion, or costochondral separation.

SPECIAL CONSIDERATIONS/COMMENTS

This test is contraindicated if there is an obvious deformity or possible lung trauma. A modification to this test is known as the Anterior/Posterior Rib Compression Test.

REFERENCE

Feng J, Hu T, Liu W, et al. The biomechanical, morphologic, and histochemical properties of the costal cartilages in children with pectus excavatum. *J Pediatr Surg.* 2001;36(12):1770-1776.

INSPIRATION/EXPIRATION BREATHING TEST

TEST POSITIONING

The subject may sit or stand. The examiner stands next to the subject.

ACTION

The subject is instructed to breathe in and out normally and then take a deep breath followed by rapid expiration.

POSITIVE FINDING

Normal breathing that is rapid and shallow is indicative of a rib fracture. Pain with deep inspiration may suggest a rib fracture, costochondral separation, or external intercostal muscle strain. Pain with forced expiration may indicate costochondral separation or internal intercostal muscle strain.

SPECIAL CONSIDERATIONS/COMMENTS

With a rib fracture or costochondral separation, there is also pain with coughing, sneezing, and torso movement. Displaced rib fractures may jeopardize the function of the lungs and should be treated as a medical emergency.

REFERENCES

Boyle RK. Cough stress rib fracture in two obstetric patients: case report and pathophysiology. *Int J Obstet Anesth*. 1998;7(1):54-58.

Karlson KA. Rib stress fractures in elite rowers. A case series and proposed mechanism. *Am J Sports Med*. 1998;26(4):516-519.

Litch JA, Tuggy M. Cough induced stress fracture and arthropathy of the ribs at extreme altitude. *Int J Sports Med*. 1998;19(3):220-222.

Potter MJ, Little C, Wilson-MacDonald J. Thoracic fracture dislocations without vertebral clinical signs. *Injury*. 2003;34(12):942-943.

Roberge RJ, Morgenstern MJ, Osborn H. Cough fracture of the ribs. *Am J Emerg Med*. 1984;2(6):513-517.

Please see videos on the accompanying website at
www.healio.com/books/specialtestsvideos

THORACIC SPINE

Section

7

Lumbar Spine

Guide to Figures

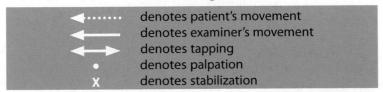

◄········ denotes patient's movement
◄——— denotes examiner's movement
◄———► denotes tapping
• denotes palpation
x denotes stabilization

Konin JG, Lebsack D, Snyder Valier AR, Isear JA Jr.
Special Tests for Orthopedic Examination, Fourth Edition (pp 165-207).
© 2016 SLACK Incorporated.

VALSALVA'S MANEUVER

TEST POSITIONING

The subject should sit. The examiner stands next to the subject.

ACTION

The examiner asks the subject to take a deep breath and hold while bearing down, as if having a bowel movement.

POSITIVE FINDING

Increased pain due to increased intrathecal pressure, which may be secondary to a space-occupying lesion, herniated disk, tumor, or osteophyte in the cervical canal, is a positive finding. Pain may be localized or referred to the corresponding dermatome.

SPECIAL CONSIDERATIONS/COMMENTS

The increased pressure may alter venous function and cause dizziness or unconsciousness. The examiner should be prepared to steady the subject. It is important to note that this test is also used to identify potential herniated discs in the lumbar spine. Increased pain in the lumbar region of the spine while performing the Valsalva's Maneuver may indicate a herniated disc. In general, this is a very general, nondescriptive, provocative test.

EVIDENCE

	Wainner et al (2003)
Study design	Diagnostic accuracy
Conditions evaluated	Cervical radiculopathy
Sample size	82
Reliability	Kappa = .69
Sensitivity	22
Specificity	94

LUMBAR SPINE

References

Childs JD. One on one. The impact of the Valsalva maneuver during resistance exercise. *Strength Cond J.* 1999;21(2):54-55.

Dyste KH, Newkirk KM. Pneumomediastinum in a high school football player: a case report. *J Athl Train.* 1998;33(4):362-364.

Folta A, Metzger BL, Therrien B. Preexisting physical activity level and cardiovascular responses across the Valsalva maneuver. *Nurs Res.* 1989;38(3):139-143.

Goldish GD, Quast JE, Blow JJ, Kuskowski MA. Postural effects on intra-abdominal pressure during Valsalva maneuver. *Arch Phys Med Rehabil.* 1994;75(3):324-327.

Kollef MH, Neelon-Kollef RA. Pulmonary embolism associated with the act of defecation. *Heart Lung.* 1991;20(5 Pt 1):451-454.

Lu Z, Metzger BL, Therrien B. Ethnic differences in physiological responses associated with the Valsalva maneuver. *Res Nurs Heath.* 1990;13(1):9-15.

Metzger BL, Therrien B. Effect of position on cardiovascular response during the Valsalva maneuver. *Nurs Res.* 1990;39(4):198-202.

Naliboff BD, Gilmore SL, Rosenthal MJ. Acute autonomic responses to postural change, Valsalva maneuver, and paced breathing in older type II diabetic men. *J Am Geriatr Soc.* 1993;41(6):648-653.

Nornhold P. Decreased cardiac output from Valsalva maneuver. *Nursing.* 1986;16(10):33.

O'Connor P, Sforzo GA, Frye P. Effect of breathing instruction on blood pressure responses during isometric exercise. *Phys Ther.* 1989;69(9):757-761.

Pierce MJ, Weesner CL, Anderson AR, Albohm MJ. Pneumomediastinum in a female track and field athlete: a case report. *J Athl Train.* 1998;33(2):168-170.

Rubinstein SM, Pool JJ, van Tulder MW, Riphagen II, de Vet HC. A systematic review of the diagnostic accuracy of provocative tests of the neck for diagnosing cervical radiculopathy. *Eur Spine J.* 2007;16(3):307-319.

Tentolouris N, Tsapogas P, Papazachos G, Katsilambros N. Corrected QT interval during the Valsalva maneuver in diabetic subjects. *Diabetes.* 2000;49(5):168.

Therrien B. Position modifies carotid artery blood flow velocity during straining. *Res Nurs Heath.* 1990;13(2):69-76.

Wainner RS, Fritz JM, Irrgang JJ, Boninger ML, Delitto A, Allison S. Reliability and diagnostic accuracy of the clinical examination and patient self-report measures for cervical radiculopathy. *Spine (Phila Pa 1976).* 2003;28(1):52-62.

Stoop Test

Test Positioning

The subject is asked to walk briskly for 1 minute.

Action

The examiner assesses for the onset of pain in the buttocks and lower limb areas. If present, the subject forward-flexes the trunk (Figure LS7-1).

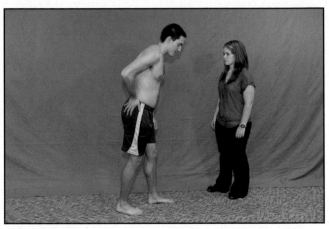

Figure LS7-1.

Positive Finding

Pain in the buttocks and lower limb areas brought on by brisk walking that is soon relieved with forward-flexing of the trunk is an indication that there is a relationship between the neurogenic intermittent claudication, posture, and walking.

Special Considerations/Comments

A positive test can be reconfirmed by positioning the patient back into trunk extension, which may reproduce the painful symptoms.

REFERENCES

Dyck P. The stoop-test in lumbar entrapment radiculopathy. *Spine (Phila Pa 1976)*. 1979;4(1):89-92.

Laessøe U, Voight M. Modification of stretch tolerance in a stooping position. *Scand J Med Sci Sports*. 2004;14(4):239-244.

Porter RW. Spinal stenosis and neurogenic claudication. *Spine (Phila Pa 1976)*. 1996;21(17):2046-2052.

HOOVER TEST

TEST POSITIONING

The subject relaxes in a supine position on the table while the examiner places both of the subject's heels into the palm of the examiner's hands (Figure LS7-2A).

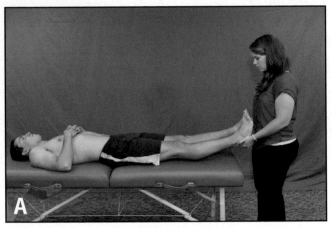

Figure LS7-2A.

ACTION

The subject is asked to perform a unilateral straight leg raise (Figure LS7-2B).

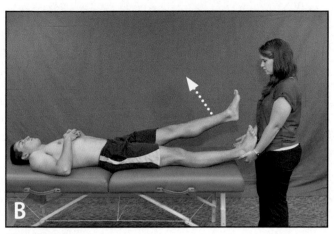

Figure LS7-2B.

LUMBAR
SPINE

POSITIVE FINDING

The inability to lift the leg may reflect a neuromuscular weakness. A positive finding is also noted when the examiner does not feel increased pressure in the palm that underlies the resting leg.

SPECIAL CONSIDERATIONS/COMMENTS

Typically, when the raised leg is weak, pressure under the resting calcaneus will increase in an attempt to lift the weak leg. When this increase in pressure is not felt, it could indicate a lack of effort by the subject. Therefore, this test should be performed on both sides to test consistency of effort.

EVIDENCE

	McWhirter et al (2011)
Study design	Cohort
Conditions evaluated	Functional weakness
Sample size	337
Reliability	Not evaluated
Sensitivity	63
Specificity	100

References

Arieff AJ. The Hoover sign: an objective sign of pain and/or weakness in the back or lower extremities. *Trans Am Neurol Assoc.* 1961;86:191.

Hoover CF. A new sign for the detection of malingering and functional paresis of the lower extremities. *JAMA.* 1908;LI(9):746-747.

Koehler PJ, Okun MS. Important observations prior to the description of the Hoover sign. *Neurology.* 2004;63(9):1693-1697.

McWhirter L, Stone J, Sandercock P, Whiteley W. Hoover's sign for the diagnosis of functional weakness: a prospective unblinded cohort study in patients with suspected stroke. *J Psychosom Res.* 2011;71(6):384-386.

Pearson CM. Differential diagnosis of neuromuscular disease by clinical evaluation. *Arch Phys Med Rehabil.* 1966;47(3):122-125.

Ziy I, Djaldetti RL, Zoldan Y, Avraham M, Melamed E. Diagnosis of "nonorganic" limb paresis by a novel objective motor assessment: the quantitative Hoover test. *J Neurol.* 1998;245(12):797-802.

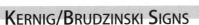

KERNIG/BRUDZINSKI SIGNS

TEST POSITIONING

The subject lies supine with his or her hands cupped behind the head. The examiner stands next to the subject.

ACTION

The subject is instructed to flex the cervical spine by lifting the head. Each hip is unilaterally flexed to no more than 90 degrees by the subject. The subject then flexes the knee to no more than 90 degrees. The opposite leg remains on the examining table (Figure LS7-3).

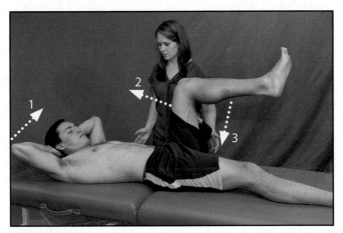

Figure LS7-3.

POSITIVE FINDING

The test is confirmed by increased pain (that is either localized or radiates into the lower extremity) with neck and hip flexion. The pain is relieved when the knee is flexed. The pain is indicative of meningeal irritation, nerve root impingement, or dural irritation that is exaggerated by elongating the spinal cord.

Special Considerations/Comments

The considerations are similar to the straight leg raise test except the neck is flexed and the hip is actively flexed. The neck flexion component of this test was developed by Kernig, and the hip flexion component was developed by Brudzinski.

Evidence

	Thomas et al (2002)	Bilavsky et al (2013)
Study design	Diagnostic accuracy	Diagnostic accuracy
Conditions evaluated	Meningitis	Meningitis
Sample size	297	86
Reliability	Not evaluated	Not evaluated
Sensitivity	Kernig sign = 5 Brudzinski sign = 5	Kernig sign = 51 Brudzinski sign = 53
Specificity	Kernig sign = 95 Brudzinski sign = 95	Kernig sign = 95 Brudzinski sign = 78

References

Bilavsky E, Leibovitz E, Elkon-Tamir E, Fruchtman Y, Ifergan G, Greenberg D. The diagnostic accuracy of the 'classic meningeal signs' in children with suspected bacterial meningitis. *Eur J Emerg Med.* 2013;20(5):361-363.

Brody IA, Wilkins RH. The signs of Kernig and Brudzinski. *Arch Neurol.* 1969;21(2):215-218.

Mehndiratta MM, Nayak R, Garg H, Kumar M, Pandey S. Appraisal of Kernig's and Brudzinski's sign in meningitis. *Ann Indian Acad Neurol.* 2013;15(4):287-288.

Pullen RL Jr. Assessing for signs of meningitis. *Nursing.* 2004;34(5):18.

Thomas KE, Hasbun R, Jekel J, Quagliarello VJ. The diagnostic accuracy of Kernig's sign, Brudzinski's sign, and nuchal rigidity in adults with suspected meningitis. *Clin Infect Dis.* 2002;35(1):46-52.

LUMBAR SPINE

Verghese A, Gallemore G. Kernig's and Brudzinski's signs revisited. *Rev Infect Dis.* 1987;9(6):1187-1192.

Ward MA, Greenwood TM, Kumar DR, Mazza JJ, Yale SH. Josef Brudzinski and Vladimir Mikhailovich Kernig: signs for diagnosing meningitis. *Clin Med Res.* 2010;8(1):13-17.

Wartenberg R. Lasègue sign and Kernig sign; historical notes. *AMA Arch Neurol Psychiatry.* 1951;66(1):58-60.

Wartenberg R. The signs of Brudzinski and of Kernig. *J Pediatr.* 1950;37(4):679-84.

90-90 STRAIGHT LEG RAISE TEST

TEST POSITIONING

The patient lies supine, stabilizing both hips at 90 degrees of flexion with both hands. The knees are bent in a relaxed position. The examiner stands next to the patient (Figure LS7-4A).

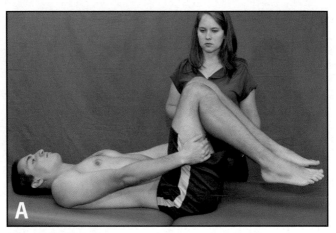

Figure LS7-4A.

ACTION

The patient is instructed to actively extend one knee at a time as much as possible (Figure LS7-4B).

POSITIVE FINDING

If the knee is flexed greater than 20 degrees, the hamstrings are considered tight.

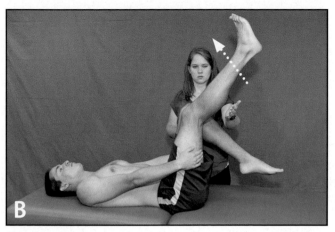

Figure LS7-4B.

Special Considerations/Comments

When assessing this test, care should always be taken to be consistent with the position of the pelvis so testing measures can be repeated with reliability.

References

Cameron DM, Bohannon RW. Relationship between active knee extension and active straight leg raise test measurements. *J Orthop Sports Phys Ther.* 1993;17(5):257-260.

Draper DO, Castro JL, Feland B, Schulthies S, Eggett D. Shortwave diathermy and prolonged stretching increase hamstring flexibility more than prolonged stretching alone. *J Orthop Sports Phys Ther.* 2004;34(1):13-20.

Gabbe BJ, Bennell KL, Wajswelner H, Finch CF. Reliability of common lower extremity musculoskeletal screening tests. *Phys Ther Sport.* 2004;5(2):90-97.

Gajdosik RL, Rieck MA, Sullivan DK, Wightman SE. Comparison of four clinical tests for assessing hamstring muscle length. *J Orthop Sports Phys Ther.* 1993;18(5):614-618.

Tafazzoli F, Lamontagne M. Mechanical behaviour of hamstring muscles in low-back pain patients and control subjects. *Clin Biomech (Bristol, Avon).* 1996;11(1):16-24.

BOWSTRING TEST (CRAM TEST)

TEST POSITIONING

The subject lies supine.

ACTION

The examiner performs a passive straight leg raise on the involved side (Figure LS7-5A). If the subject reports radiating pain with the straight leg raised, the examiner then flexes the subject's knee to approximately 20 degrees in an attempt to reduce painful symptoms (Figure LS7-5B). The examiner then applies pressure to the popliteal area in an attempt to reproduce the radicular pain.

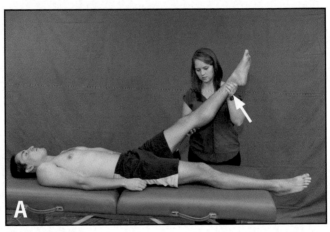

Figure LS7-5A.

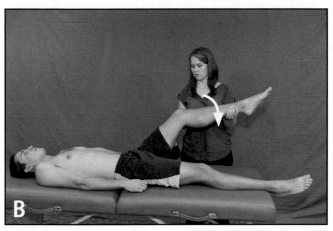

Figure LS7-5B.

POSITIVE FINDING

Painful radicular reproduction following popliteal compression indicates tension on the sciatic nerve.

SPECIAL CONSIDERATIONS/COMMENTS

It is important for the examiner to maintain the same degree of the subject's hip flexion when flexion of the knee is performed.

EVIDENCE

	Supik and Broom (1994)
Study design	Diagnostic accuracy
Conditions evaluated	Lumbar disc herniation
Sample size	50
Reliability	Not evaluated
Sensitivity	69
Specificity	Not evaluated

REFERENCES

Herron LD, Pheasant HC. Bilateral laminotomy and discectomy for segmental lumbar disc disease. Decompression with stability. *Spine (Phila Pa 1976)*. 1983;8(1):86-97.

Supik LF, Broom MJ. Sciatic tension signs and lumbar disc herniation. *Spine (Phila Pa 1976)*. 1994;19(9):1066-1069.

Sitting Root Test

Test Positioning

The subject sits with the hip and knee flexed to 90 degrees and the cervical spine in flexion.

Action

The subject actively extends the knee (Figure LS7-6A).

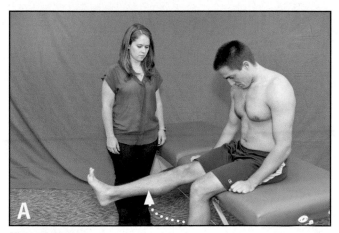

Figure LS7-6A.

Positive Finding

The subject who arches backward and/or complains of pain in the regions of the buttocks, posterior thigh, and calf during knee extension demonstrates a positive finding for possible sciatic nerve pain.

SPECIAL CONSIDERATIONS/COMMENTS

This test can be reproduced with the examiner passively extending the subject's knee. True sciatic pain should still cause the subject to react. However, if the examiner's actions distract the subject from being aware of the area being tested, the subject may respond differently. For example, if the examiner stabilized and took note of the foot during extension of the knee, the subject may be unaware that the examiner is really testing for sciatic tension (Figure LS7-6B).

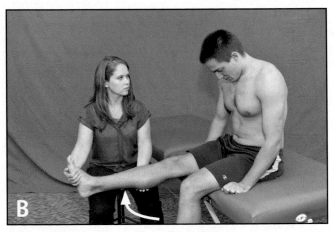

Figure LS7-6B.

REFERENCE

Lew PC, Briggs CA. Relationship between the cervical component of the slump test and change in hamstring muscle tension. *Man Ther.* 1997;2(2):98-105.

Unilateral Straight Leg Raise Test (Lasègue Test)

Test Positioning

The subject is supine with both hips and knees extended. The examiner is standing with the distal hand around the subject's heel and the proximal hand on the subject's distal thigh (anteriorly) to maintain knee extension.

Action

With the subject completely relaxed, the examiner slowly raises the test leg until pain or tightness is noted (Figure LS7-7A). The examiner slowly lowers the leg until the pain or tightness resolves and then dorsiflexes the ankle (Figure LS7-7B) and instructs the subject to flex the neck (Figure LS7-7C).

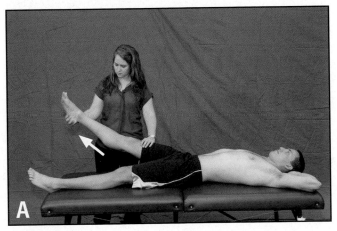

Figure LS7-7A.

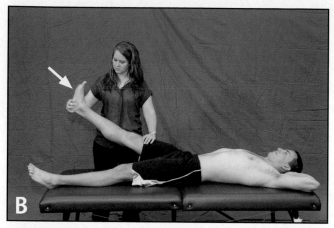

Figure LS7-7B.

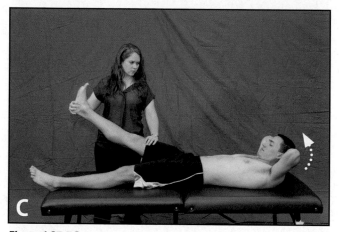

Figure LS7-7C.

POSITIVE FINDING

Leg and/or low back pain occurring with dorsiflexion and/or neck flexion is indicative of dural involvement. A lack of pain reproduction with dorsiflexion and/or neck flexion is indicative of either hamstring tightness or possible lumbar spine or sacroiliac joint involvement. Additionally, pain occurring at hip flexion angles greater than 70 degrees is indicative of lumbar spine or sacroiliac joint involvement. If the latter is determined, proceed to the bilateral straight leg raise test to differentiate between lumbar spine and sacroiliac joint involvement.

SPECIAL CONSIDERATIONS/COMMENTS

The subject must be completely relaxed because contraction of the hip flexor muscles could increase the stress placed on the lumbar spine and sacroiliac joint, thus creating false-positive findings. Additionally, during the Unilateral Straight Leg Raise Test, pain may be noted in the contralateral leg and/or lumbar spine. This finding should be referred to as a positive Crossed Straight Leg Raise Test.

EVIDENCE

	Devillé et al (2000)	Gabbe et al (2004)	Majlesi et al (2008)
Study design	Meta-analysis	Reliability	Case control
Conditions evaluated	Herniated discs	Screening	Lumbar disc herniation
Study number	11		
Sample size		15	75
Reliability	Not evaluated	ICC = .91	Not evaluated
Sensitivity	91	Not evaluated	52
Specificity	26	Not evaluated	89

REFERENCES

Cameron DM, Bohannon RW, Owen SV. Influence of hip position on measurements of straight leg raise test. *J Orthop Sports Phys Ther.* 1994;19(3):168-172.

Chow R, Adams R, Herbert R. Straight leg raise test high reliability is not a motor memory artefact. *Aust J Physiother.* 1994;40(2):107-111.

Devillé WL, van der Windt DA, Dzaferagić A, Bezemer PD, Bouter LM. The test of Lasègue: systematic review of the accuracy in diagnosing herniated discs. *Spine (Phila Pa 1976).* 2000;25(9):1140-1147.

Gabbe BJ, Bennell KL, Wajswelner H, Finch CF. Reliability of common lower extremity musculoskeletal screening tests. *Phys Ther Sport.* 2004;5(2):90-97.

Idota H, Yoshida T. Clinical significance of the straight-leg-raising test. *Nihon Seikeigeka Gakkai Zasshi.* 1991;65(11):1035-1044.

Iglesias-Casarrubios P, Alday-Anzola R, Ruíz-López P, Gómez-López P, Cruz-Bértolo J, Lobato RD. Lasegue's test as prognostic factor for patients undergoing lumbar disc surgery [article in Spanish]. *Neurocirugia (Astur).* 2004;15(2):138-143.

Kohlboeck G, Greimel KV, Piotrowski WP, et al. Prognosis of multifactorial outcome in lumbar discectomy: a prospective longitudinal study investigating patients with disc prolapse. *Clin J Pain.* 2004;20(6):455-461.

Łebkowski WJ. Presence and intensity of the Lasegue sign in relation to the site lumbar intervertebral disc herniation [article in Polish]. *Chir Narzadow Ruchu Ortop Pol.* 2002;67(3):265-268.

Majlesi J, Togay H, Unalan H, Toprak S. The sensitivity and specificity of the Slump and the Straight Leg Raising tests in patients with lumbar disc herniation. *J Clin Rheumatol.* 2008;14(2):87-91.

Mens JM, Vleeming A, Snijders CJ, Koes BW, Stam HJ. Reliability and validity of the active straight leg raise test in posterior pelvic pain since pregnancy. *Spine (Phila Pa 1976).* 2001;26(10):1167-1171.

Meszaros TF, Olson R, Kulig K, Creighton D, Czarnecki E. Effect of 10%, 30%, and 60% body weight traction on the straight leg raise test of symptomatic patients with low back pain. *J Orthop Sports Phys Ther.* 2000;30(10):595-601.

Neto T, Jacobsohn L, Carita AI, Oliveira R. Reliability of the Active Knee Extension Test and the Straight Leg Raise Test in subjects with flexibility deficits [published online ahead of print October 30, 2014]. *J Sport Rehabil.* doi:10.1123/jsr.2014-0220.

Wartenberg R. Lasègue sign and Kernig sign; historical notes. *AMA Arch Neurol Psychiatry.* 1951;66(1):58-60.

BILATERAL STRAIGHT LEG RAISE TEST

TEST POSITIONING

The subject lies supine with both hips and knees extended. The examiner is standing with the distal hand or forearm around or under the subject's heels and the proximal hand on the subject's distal thighs (anteriorly) to maintain knee extension.

ACTION

With the subject completely relaxed, slowly raise the legs until pain or tightness is noted (Figure LS7-8).

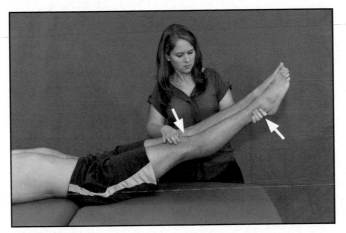

Figure LS7-8.

POSITIVE FINDING

Low back pain occurring at hip flexion angles less than 70 degrees is indicative of sacroiliac joint involvement. Low back pain occurring at hip flexion angles greater than 70 degrees is indicative of lumbar spine involvement.

LUMBAR
SPINE

188   Section 7

SPECIAL CONSIDERATIONS/COMMENTS

The examiner must use proper body mechanics when performing this test to avoid injury secondary to lifting the weight of both legs. The examiner should also note any excessive pelvic motion that may indicate the subject's discomfort and/or mechanical compensation associated with the test.

REFERENCES

Baltaci G, Un N, Tunay V, Besler A, Gerçeker S. Comparison of three different sit and reach tests for measurement of hamstring flexibility in female university students. Br J Sports Med. 2003;37(1):59-61.

Hunt DG, Zuberbier OA, Kozlowski AJ, et al. Reliability of the lumbar flexion, lumbar extension, and passive straight leg raise test in normal populations embedded within a complete physical examination. Spine (Phila Pa 1976). 2001;26(24):2714-2718.

Mens JM, Vleeming A, Snijders CJ, Koes BW, Stam HJ. Validity of the active straight leg raise test for measuring disease severity in patients with posterior pelvic pain after pregnancy. Spine (Phila Pa 1976). 2002;27(2):196-200.

O'Sullivan PB, Beales DJ, Beetham JA, et al. Altered motor control strategies in subjects with sacroiliac joint pain during the active straight-leg-raise test. Spine (Phila Pa 1976). 2002;27(1):E1-E8.

Rade M, Könönen M, Vanninen R, et al. 2014 young investigator award winner: In vivo magnetic resonance imaging measurement of spinal cord displacement in the thoracolumbar region of asymptomatic subjects: part 2: comparison between unilateral and bilateral straight leg raise tests. Spine (Phila Pa 1976). 39(16):1294-1300.

Rebain R, Baxter GD, McDonough S. The passive straight leg raising test in the diagnosis and treatment of lumbar disc herniation: a survey of United Kingdom osteopathic opinion and clinical practice. Spine (Phila Pa 1976). 2003;28(15):1717-1724.

WELL STRAIGHT LEG RAISE TEST (CROSSED STRAIGHT LEG RAISE)

TEST POSITIONING

The subject lies supine on a table. The examiner places one hand on the anterior aspect of the uninvolved leg slightly superior to the knee and the other hand around the heel of the ipsilateral calcaneus.

ACTION

The examiner passively flexes the subject's uninvolved hip while maintaining the knee in an extended position (Figure LS7-9).

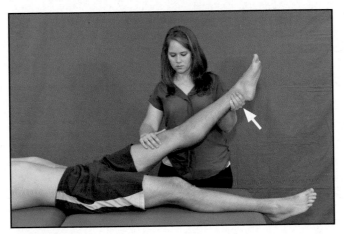

Figure LS7-9.

LUMBAR SPINE

POSITIVE FINDING

Complaints of pain on the involved side indicate a positive test and may be related to vertebral disk damage.

Special Considerations/Comments

This test was first described by Fajersztajn but is also known as a prostrate leg raising test, Lhermitte's test, or a cross-over sign. When this test is performed, a dural stretch is applied to both sides of the lower extremity. Therefore, complaints of pain may be noted in a radicular manner.

Evidence

	Devillé et al (2000)
Study design	Systematic review
Conditions evaluated	Herniated discs
Study number	6
Reliability	Not evaluated
Sensitivity	29
Specificity	88

References

Devillé WL, van der Windt DA, Dzaferagić A, Bezemer PD, Bouter LM. The test of Lasègue: systematic review of the accuracy in diagnosing herniated discs. *Spine (Phila Pa 1976)*. 2000;25(9):1140-1147.

Gajdosik RL, Rieck MA, Sullivan DK, Wightman SE. Comparison of four clinical tests for assessing hamstring muscle length. *J Orthop Sports Phys Ther*. 1993;18(5):614-618.

Jönsson B, Strömqvist B. Significance of a persistent positive straight leg raising test after lumbar disc surgery. *J Neurosurg*. 1999;91(1 Suppl):50-53.

Jönsson B, Strömqvist B. The straight leg raising test and the severity of symptoms in lumbar disc herniation. A preoperative evaluation. *Spine (Phila Pa 1976)*. 1995;20(1):27-30.

Rebain R, Baxter GD, McDonough S. The passive straight leg raising test in the diagnosis and treatment of lumbar disc herniation: a survey of United Kingdom osteopathic opinion and clinical practice. *Spine (Phila Pa 1976)*. 2003;28(15):1717-1724.

Woodhall B, Hayes GJ. The well-leg raising test of Fajersztajn in the diagnosis of ruptured lumbar intervertebral disc. *J Bone Joint Surg Am*. 1950;32A(4):786-792.

LUMBAR SPINE

SLUMP TEST

TEST POSITIONING

The subject sits on the end of the table and leans forward while the examiner holds the head and chin upright (Figure LS7-10A).

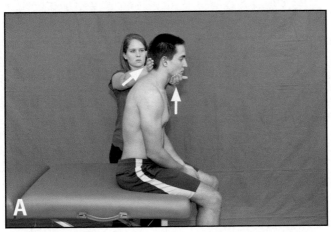

Figure LS7-10A.

ACTION

Any symptomatic changes reported by the subject are noted. The examiner then flexes the subject's neck and assesses for any changes in symptoms (Figure LS7-10B). If no changes are noted, the examiner passively extends one of the subject's knees (Figure LS7-10C). Again, symptomatic changes are assessed. With no noted changes, the examiner then passively dorsiflexes the subject's ankle while the knee remains extended (Figure LS7-10D). The subject is then returned to the original "slump" position and the test is repeated for the other leg.

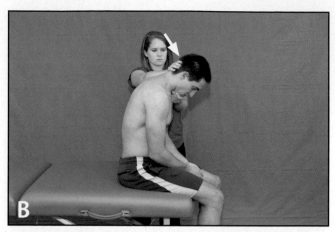

Figure LS7-10B.

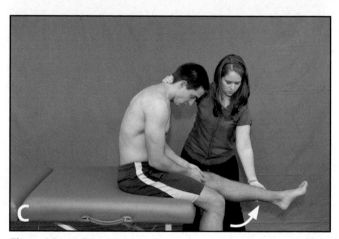

Figure LS7-10C.

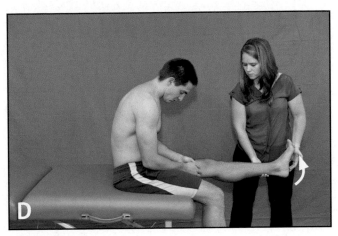

Figure LS7-10D.

POSITIVE FINDING

A complaint of sciatic-type pain or any reproduction of symptoms is indicative of a positive test.

SPECIAL CONSIDERATIONS/COMMENTS

The examiner should note the location of the symptomatic changes because this is often the site of a dural stretch. Others have described this test whereby the subject actively moves the knee and ankle as opposed to passive movement.

EVIDENCE

	Gabbe et al (2004)	Majlesi et al (2008)
Study design	Reliability	Case control
Conditions evaluated	Screening	Lumbar disc herniation
Sample size	15	75
Reliability	ICC = .92	Not evaluated
Sensitivity	Not evaluated	84
Specificity	Not evaluated	83

REFERENCES

Gabbe BJ, Bennell KL, Wajswelner H, Finch CF. Reliability of common lower extremity musculoskeletal screening tests. *Phys Ther Sport.* 2004;5(2):90-97.

Johnson EK, Chiarello CM. The slump test: the effects of head and lower extremity position on knee extension. *J Orthop Sports Phys Ther.* 1997;26(6):310-317.

Lew PC, Briggs CA. Relationship between the cervical component of the slump test and change in hamstring muscle tension. *Man Ther.* 1997;2(2):98-105.

Majlesi J, Togay H, Unalan H, Toprak S. The sensitivity and specificity of the Slump and the Straight Leg Raising tests in patients with lumbar disc herniation. *J Clin Rheumatol.* 2008;14(2):87-91.

Pahor S, Toppenberg R. An investigation of neural tissue involvement in ankle inversion sprains. *Man Ther.* 1996;1(4):192-197.

Stankovic R, Johnell O, Maly P, Willner S. Use of lumbar extension, slump test, physical and neurological examination in the evaluation of patients with suspected herniated nucleus pulposus. A prospective clinical study. *Man Ther.* 1999;4(1):25-32.

Webright WG, Randolph BJ, Perrin DH. Comparison of nonballistic active knee extension in neural slump position and static stretch techniques on hamstring flexibility. *J Orthop Sports Phys Ther.* 1997;26(1):7-13.

White MA, Pape KE. The slump test. *Am J Occup Ther.* 1992;46(3):271-274.

THOMAS TEST

TEST POSITIONING

The subject lies supine with both knees fully flexed against the chest and the buttocks near the table edge. The examiner stands with one hand on the subject's lumbar spine or iliac crest to monitor lumbar lordosis or pelvic tilt, respectively (Figure LS7-11A).

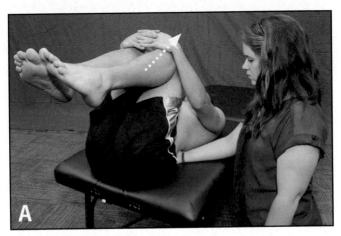

Figure LS7-11A.

ACTION

The subject slowly lowers the test leg until it is fully relaxed or until either anterior pelvic tilting or an increase in lumbar lordosis occurs (Figure LS7-11B).

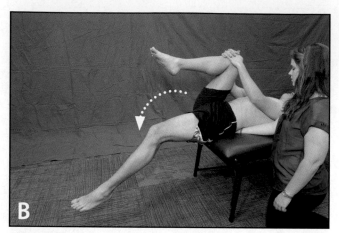

Figure LS7-11B.

LUMBAR SPINE

POSITIVE FINDING

A lack of hip extension with knee flexion greater than 45 degrees is indicative of iliopsoas muscle tightness. Full hip extension with knee flexion less than 45 degrees is indicative of rectus femoris muscle tightness. A lack of hip extension with knee flexion less than 45 degrees is indicative of iliopsoas and rectus femoris muscle tightness. Hip external rotation during any of the previous scenarios is indicative of iliotibial band tightness.

SPECIAL CONSIDERATIONS/COMMENTS

Increases in anterior pelvic tilt and lumbar lordosis must be eliminated to prevent false-negative findings. To further confirm this assessment, the examiner can simply apply pressure on the lower leg in an effort to lower it back to the table. A return of lumbar lordosis will indicate a positive finding.

EVIDENCE

	Gabbe et al (2004)
Study design	Reliability study
Conditions evaluated	Screening
Sample size	15
Reliability	ICC = .63 to .75
Sensitivity	Not evaluated
Specificity	Not evaluated

REFERENCES

Barlett MD, Wolf LS, Shurtleff DB, Stahell LT. Hip flexion contractures: a comparison of measurement methods. *Arch Phys Med Rehabil.* 1985;66(9):620-625.

Eland DC, Singleton TN, Conaster RR, et al. The "iliacus test": new information for the evaluation of hip extension dysfunction. *J Am Osteopath Assoc.* 2002;102(3):130-142.

Gabbe BJ, Bennell KL, Wajswelner H, Finch CF. Reliability of common lower extremity musculoskeletal screening tests. *Phys Ther Sport.* 2004;5(2):90-97.

Harvey D. Assessment of the flexibility of elite athletes using the modified Thomas test. *Br J Sports Med.* 1998;32(1)68-70.

Harvey DM. Flexibility of elite athletes using the modified Thomas test. *Med Sci Sport Exerc.* 1997;29(5):271.

Koyama H, Murakami K, Suzuki T, Suzaki K. Phenol block for hip flexor muscle spasticity under ultrasonic monitoring. *Arch Phys Med Rehabil.* 1992;73(11):1040-1043.

Lee LW, Kerrigan D, Casey MD, Della Croce U. Dynamic implications of hip flexion contractures. *Am J Phys Med Rehabil.* 1997;76(6):502-508.

Margo K, Drezner J, Motzkin D. Evaluation and management of hip pain: an algorithmic approach. *J Fam Pract.* 2003;52(8):607-617.

Narvani AA, Tsiridis E, Kendall S, Chaudhuri R, Thomas P. A preliminary report on prevalence of acetabular labrum tears in sports patients with groin pain. *Knee Surg Sports Traumatol Arthrosc.* 2003;11(6):403-408.

Reiman MP, Goode AP, Hegedus EJ, Cook CE, Wright AA. Diagnostic accuracy of clinical tests of the hip: a systematic review with meta-analysis. *Br J Sports Med.* 2013;47(14):893-902.

LUMBAR SPINE

Schache AG, Blanch PD, Murphy AT. Relation of anterior pelvic tilt during running to clinical and kinematic measures of hip extension. *Br J Sports Med.* 2000;34(4):279-283.

Tyler T, Zook L, Brittis D, Gleim G. A new pelvic tilt detection device: roentgenographic validation and application to assessment of hip motion in professional ice hockey players. *J Orthop Sports Phys Ther.* 1996;24(5):303-308.

Winters MV, Blake CG, Trost JS, et al. Passive versus active stretching of hip flexor muscles in subjects with limited hip extension: a randomized clinical trial. *Phys Ther.* 2004;84(9):800-807.

Young W, Clothier P, Otago L, Bruce L, Liddell D. Acute effects of static stretching on hip flexor and quadriceps flexibility, range of motion and foot speed in kicking a football. *J Sci Med Sport.* 2004;7(1):23-31.

Spring Test

Test Positioning

The subject lies prone and the examiner stands with the thumb (Figure LS7-12A) or hypothenar eminence (specifically the pisiform) over the spinous process of a lumbar vertebra (Figure LS7-12B).

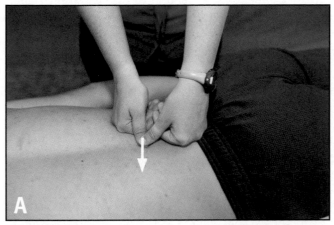

Figure LS7-12A.

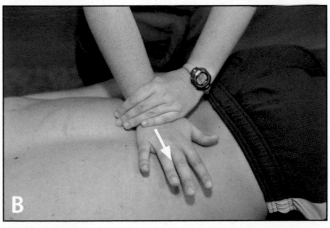

Figure LS7-12B.

ACTION

Apply a downward "springing" force through the spinous process of each vertebra to assess posterior-anterior motion. This action should be repeated for each transverse process to assess rotary motion.

POSITIVE FINDING

Increases or decreases in motion at one vertebra compared to another are indicative of hypermobility or hypomobility, respectively.

SPECIAL CONSIDERATIONS/COMMENTS

Rotational accessory movement can be compared at each level by performing this test to the transverse process on each side of one vertebral level.

REFERENCES

Billis EV, Foster NE, Wright CC. Reproducibility and repeatability: errors of three groups of physiotherapists in locating spinal levels by palpation. *Man Ther.* 2003;8(4):223-232.

Chansirinukor W, Lee M, Latimer J. Contribution of pelvic rotation to lumbar posteroanterior movement. *Man Ther.* 2001;6(4):242-249.

Edmondston SJ, Allison GT, Gregg CD, Purden SM, Svansson GR, Watson AE. Effect of position on the posteroanterior stiffness of the lumbar spine. *Man Ther.* 1998;3(1):21-26.

Latimer J, Lee M, Adams R. The effect of training with feedback on physiotherapy students' ability to judge lumbar stiffness. *Man Ther.* 1996;1(5):266-270.

Nyland J, Johnson D. Collegiate football players display more active cervical spine mobility than high school football players. *J Athl Train.* 2004;39(2):146-150.

Petty NJ. The effect of posteroanterior mobilisation on sagittal mobility of the lumbar spine. *Man Ther.* 2000;1(1):25-29.

Petty NJ, Maher C, Latimer J, Lee M. Manual examination of accessory movements—seeking R1. *Man Ther.* 2002;7(1):39-43.

Shirley D, Ellis E, Lee M. The response of posteroanterior lumbar stiffness to repeated loading. *Man Ther.* 2002;7(1):19-25.

TRENDELENBURG'S TEST

TEST POSITIONING

The subject stands on one lower extremity (Figure LS7-13A).

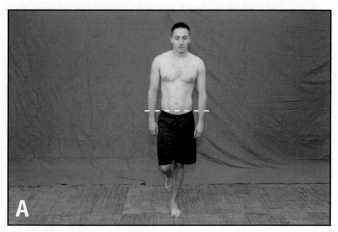

Figure LS7-13A.

ACTION

The subject remains in this position for approximately 10 seconds and then switches extremities.

POSITIVE FINDING

A positive finding is seen when the pelvis on the unsupported side drops noticeably lower than the pelvis on the supported side (Figure LS7-13B). This indicates a weakness of the gluteus medius muscle on the supported side. Figures LS7-13C and LS7-13D show the posterior view.

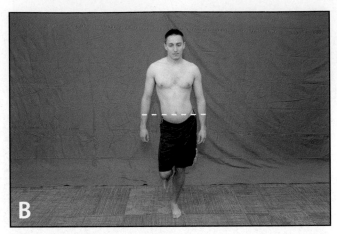

Figure LS7-13B.

SPECIAL CONSIDERATIONS/COMMENTS

With a negative test, the gluteus medius on the supported side will perform a reverse action because the supported femur is stabilized. This will allow for the unsupported pelvis to remain level with the supported pelvis. With a weak gluteus medius on the supported side, the unsupported pelvis drops as the muscle fatigues. This test may also indicate an unstable hip on the supported side.

EVIDENCE

	Reiman et al (2013)
Study design	Meta-analysis
Conditions evaluated	Gluteal tendinopathy
Study number	3
Sample size	78
Reliability	Not evaluated
Sensitivity	61
Specificity	92

LUMBAR SPINE

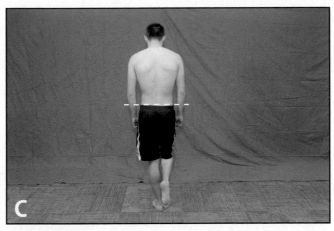

Figure LS7-13C.

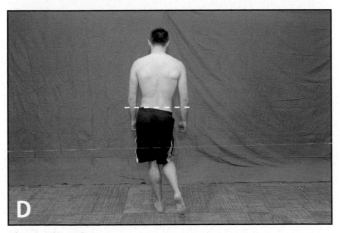

Figure LS7-13D.

REFERENCES

Asayama I, Naito M, Fujisawa M, Kambe T. Relationship between radiographic measurements of reconstructed hip joint position and the Trendelenburg sign. *J Arthroplasty.* 2002;17(6):747-751.

Bird PA, Oakley SP, Shnier R, Kirkham BW. Prospective evaluation of magnetic resonance imaging and physical examination findings in patients with greater trochanteric pain syndrome. *Arthritis Rheum.* 2001;44(9):2138-2145.

Hardcastle P, Nade S. The significance of the Trendelenburg test. *J Bone Joint Surg Br.* 1985;67(5):741-746.

Reiman MP, Goode AP, Hegedus EJ, Cook CE, Wright AA. Diagnostic accuracy of clinical tests of the hip: a systematic review with meta-analysis. *Br J Sports Med.* 2013;47(14):893-902.

Trendelenburg F. Trendelenburg's test: 1895. *Clin Orthop Relat Res.* 1998;(355):3-7.

Vasudevan PN, Vaidyalingam KV, Nair PB. Can Trendelenburg's sign be positive if the hip is normal? *J Bone Joint Surg Br.* 1997;79(3):462-466.

Youdas JW, Madson TJ, Hollman JH. Usefulness of the Trendelenburg test for identification of patients with hip joint osteoarthritis. *Physiother Theory Pract.* 2010;26(3):184-194.

LUMBAR SPINE

STORK STANDING TEST

TEST POSITIONING

The subject stands on one leg with the sole of the nonweight-bearing foot resting on the medial aspect of the knee of the weight-bearing limb (Figure LS7-14A).

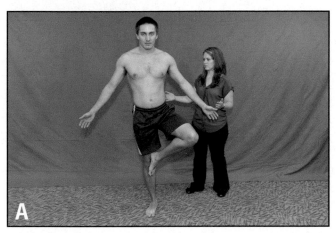

Figure LS7-14A.

ACTION

The subject maintains balance on one leg and then simultaneously performs a slight lumbar extension movement (Figure LS7-14B). The test is repeated bilaterally.

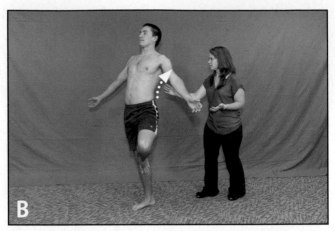

Figure LS7-14B.

POSITIVE FINDING

Complaints of pain in the lumbar region may be related to the pars interarticularis region, which is sometimes associated with spondylolysis.

SPECIAL CONSIDERATIONS/COMMENTS

This test is also referred to as the One-Leg Standing Lumbar Extension Test. The examiner should assess the level of each pelvis during the test. Changes in the pelvic levels related to gluteus medius muscle weakness may present to the examiner as a false indicator of poor proprioception. There is no ideal time frame for the length of maintained one-legged balance. The examiner should note any bilateral discrepancies that exist.

REFERENCES

Margo K, Drezner J, Motzkin D. Evaluation and management of hip pain: an algorithmic approach. *J Fam Pract.* 2003;52(8):607-617.

Narvani AA, Tsiridis E, Kendall S, Chaudhuri R, Thomas P. A preliminary report on prevalence of acetabular labrum tears in sports patients with groin pain. *Knee Surg Sports Traumatol Arthrosc.* 2003;11(6):403-408.

Peltenburg AL, Erich WB, Bernink MJ, Huisveld IA. Selection of talented female gymnasts, aged 8 to 11, on the basis of motor abilities with special reference to balance: a retrospective study. *Int J Sports Med.* 1982;3(1):37-42.

Schache AG, Blanch PD, Murphy AT. Relation of anterior pelvic tilt during running to clinical and kinematic measures of hip extension. *Br J Sports Med.* 2000;34(4):279-283.

Tyler T, Zook L, Brittis D, Gleim G. A new pelvic tilt detection device: roentgenographic validation and application to assessment of hip motion in professional ice hockey players. *J Orthop Sports Phys Ther.* 1996;24(5):303-308.

Winters MV, Blake CG, Trost JS, et al. Passive versus active stretching of hip flexor muscles in subjects with limited hip extension: a randomized clinical trial. *Phys Ther.* 2004;84(9):800-807.

Young W, Clothier P, Otago L, Bruce L, Liddell D. Acute effects of static stretching on hip flexor and quadriceps flexibility, range of motion and foot speed in kicking a football. *J Sci Med Sport.* 2004;7(1):23-31.

Please see videos on the accompanying website at
www.healio.com/books/specialtestsvideos

Section
8

Sacral Spine

Guide to Figures

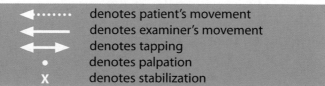

◀······· denotes patient's movement
◀────── denotes examiner's movement
◀─────▶ denotes tapping
• denotes palpation
X denotes stabilization

Konin JG, Lebsack D, Snyder Valier AR, Isear JA Jr.
Special Tests for Orthopedic Examination, Fourth Edition (pp 209-235).
© 2016 SLACK Incorporated.

Sacroiliac (SI) Joint Fixation Test

Test Positioning 1

The subject stands with the SI joint exposed. The examiner stands behind the subject with the thumbs over the posterior superior iliac spines (PSIS) (Figure SS8-1A).

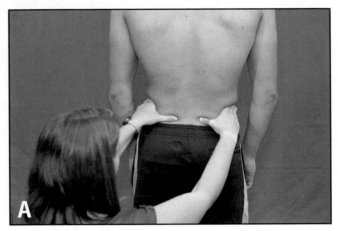

Figure SS8-1A.

Action 1

The examiner should note whether the PSIS are level.

Positive Finding 1

If the posterior iliac spines are not level, the SI joints are asymmetrical, indicating fixation on one side or the other.

Special Considerations/Comments 1

Having the subject actively flex one hip and then comparing the level of the PSIS on each side has been described as a Gillet test. Decreased or minimal inferior movement of the SI joint on the flexed side indicates a hypomobile joint.

	Levangie (1999)
Study design	Cross-sectional
Conditions evaluated	Low back pain
Sample size	288
Reliability	ICC = .70
Sensitivity	Not evaluated
Specificity	Not evaluated

Test Positioning 2

The examiner then places one thumb over the PSIS on the right or left side, and the other thumb over the S2 spinous process. Repeat on the other side (Figure SS8-1B).

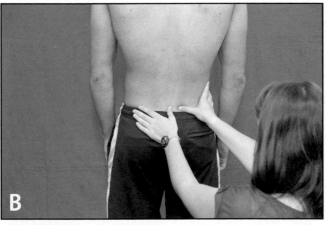

Figure SS8-1B.

Action 2

The subject is then instructed to actively flex each hip one at a time with the knee bent to 90 degrees. Compare to the other side (Figure SS8-1C).

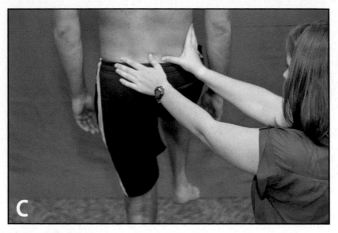

Figure SS8-1C.

Positive Finding 2

When the subject flexes each hip, the thumb over the posterior superior iliac spine should drop relative to the spinous process. If there is no change or the thumb moves superiorly, hypomobility is indicated.

Test Positioning 3

The examiner may then leave the one thumb over the sacral spinous process and move the other thumb to the ischial tuberosity. Repeat on the other side (Figure SS8-1D).

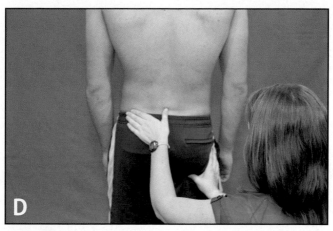

Figure SS8-1D.

ACTION 3

The subject is instructed to again actively flex one hip at a time with the knee bent to 90 degrees. Compare to the other side (Figure SS8-1E).

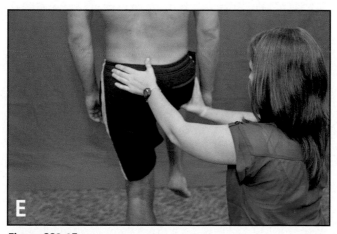

Figure SS8-1E.

POSITIVE FINDING 3

When the subject again flexes each hip, the thumb over the ischial tuberosity should move inferiorly. If the thumb moves superiorly, hypomobility is indicated.

SPECIAL CONSIDERATIONS/COMMENTS 3

Some authors have referred to this series of tests as the hip flexion test. Essentially, the same movement is being performed and the difference in assessment is based on the landmarks that are being palpated and observed for movement patterns.

REFERENCES

Levangie PK. Four clinical tests of sacroiliac joint dysfunction: the association of test results with innominate torsion among patients with and without low back pain. *Phys Ther.* 1999;79(11):1043-1057.

van der Wurff P, Meyne W, Hagmeijer RH. Clinical tests of the sacroiliac joint. *Man Ther.* 2000;5(2):89-96.

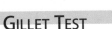

GILLET TEST

TEST POSITIONING

The subject stands while the examiner palpates the PSIS bilaterally.

ACTION

The subject flexes one hip and brings the knee to the chest while the examiner maintains palpation to each PSIS and assesses overall SI movement (Figure SS8-2A).

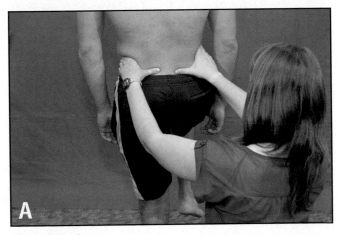

Figure SS8-2A.

POSITIVE FINDING

A positive sign is noted if the PSIS on the ipsilateral side of the knee being flexed does not move or moves minimally in the inferior direction (Figure SS8-2B).

SACRAL
SPINE

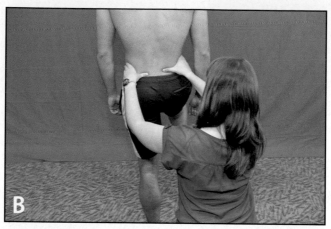

Figure SS8-2B.

SPECIAL CONSIDERATIONS/COMMENTS

The PSIS on the side of the hip being flexed should move slightly anteriorly during active hip flexion.

EVIDENCE

	van der Wurff et al (2000)	Szadek et al (2009)
Study design	Systematic review	Systematic review
Conditions evaluated	SI joint mobility	SI joint pain
Study number	6	1
Reliability	Kappa = .02 to .22	Not evaluated
Sensitivity	Not evaluated	43
Specificity	Not evaluated	68

References

Carmichael JP. Inter- and intraexaminer reliability of palpation for sacroiliac joint dysfunction. *J Manipulative Physiol Ther.* 1987;10(4):164-171.

Dreyfuss P, Dryer S, Griffin J, Hoffman J, Walsh N. Positive sacroiliac screening tests in asymptomatic adults. *Spine (Phila Pa 1976).* 1994;19(10):1138-1143.

Levangie PK. Four clinical tests of sacroiliac joint dysfunction: the association of test results with innominate torsion among patients with and without low back pain. *Phys Ther.* 1999;79(11):1043-1057.

Meijne W, van Neerbos K, Aufdemkampe G, van der Wurff P. Intraexaminer and interexaminer reliability of the Gillet test. *J Manipulative Physiol Ther.* 1999;22(1):4-9.

Szadek KM, van der Wurff P, van Tulder MW, Zuurmond WW, Perez RS. Diagnostic validity of criteria for sacroiliac joint pain: a systematic review. *J Pain.* 2009;10(4):354-368.

van der Wurff P, Hagmeijer RH, Meyne W. Clinical tests of the sacroiliac joint. A systematic methodological review. Part 1: Reliability. *Man Ther.* 2000;5(1):30-36.

SACROILIAC (SI) JOINT STRESS TEST

TEST POSITIONING 1

The subject lies supine. The examiner stands next to the subject and, with the arms crossed, places the heel of both hands on the subject's anterior superior iliac spines (Figure SS8-3A).

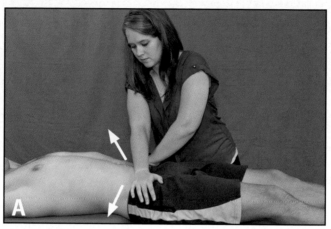

Figure SS8-3A.

ACTION 1

The examiner applies outward and downward pressure with the heel of the hands.

POSITIVE FINDING 1

Unilateral pain at the SI joint or in the gluteal or leg region indicates an anterior SI ligament sprain.

SPECIAL CONSIDERATIONS/COMMENTS 1

The subject may complain of pain that could be related to SI joint compression.

EVIDENCE

	van der Wurff et al (2000)	Szadek et al (2009)
Study design	Systematic review	Systematic review
Conditions evaluated	SI joint pain	SI joint pain
Study number	3	2
Reliability	Kappa = .36 to .69	Not evaluated
Sensitivity	Not evaluated	26 to 60
Specificity	Not evaluated	73 to 81

TEST POSITIONING 2

The subject lies on the side. The examiner stands next to the subject and places both hands, one on top of the other, directly over the subject's iliac crest. Repeat on the other side (Figure SS8-3B).

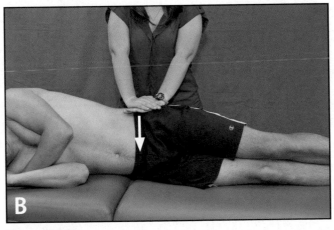

Figure SS8-3B.

ACTION 2

The examiner applies downward pressure. Compare to the other side.

POSITIVE FINDING 2

Increased pain or pressure is indicative of SI joint pathology, possibly involving the posterior SI ligaments.

SPECIAL CONSIDERATIONS/COMMENTS 2

The subject may complain of pain that could be related to SI joint distraction or gapping. This positioning is also referred to as the Compression Provocation Test.

EVIDENCE

	van der Wurff et al (2000)	Szadek et al (2009)
Study design	Systematic review	Systematic review
Conditions evaluated	SI joint pain	SI joint pain
Study number	4	2
Reliability	Kappa = .16 to .77	Not evaluated
Sensitivity	Not evaluated	60 to 69
Specificity	Not evaluated	69 to 70

TEST POSITIONING 3

The subject lies supine. The examiner places both hands on the lateral aspect of the subject's iliac crests (Figure SS8-3C).

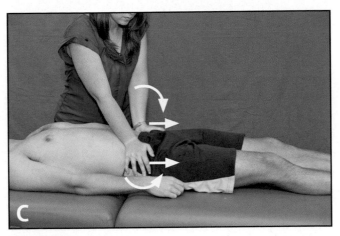

Figure SS8-3C.

ACTION 3

The examiner applies inward and downward pressure.

POSITIVE FINDING 3

Increased pain or pressure is indicative of SI joint pathology, possibly involving the posterior SI ligaments.

SPECIAL CONSIDERATIONS/COMMENTS 3

The subject may complain of pain that could be related to SI joint distraction or gapping.

Test Positioning 4

The subject lies prone. The examiner places both hands, one on top of the other, over the subject's sacrum (Figure SS8-3D).

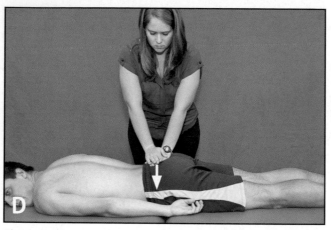

Figure SS8-3D.

Action 4

The examiner applies downward pressure, creating a shear of the sacrum on the ilium.

Positive Finding 4

Pain at the SI joint is indicative of SI joint pathology.

Special Considerations/Comments 4

The subject may complain of pain that could be related to SI joint compression. Test positioning 4 may also be referred to as the Sacral Thrust Provocation Test.

Sacral Spine   223

EVIDENCE

	van der Wurff et al (2000)	Szadek et al (2009)
Study design	Systematic review	Systematic review
Conditions evaluated	SI joint pain	SI joint pain
Study number	2	2
Reliability	Kappa = .30 to .32	Not evaluated
Sensitivity	Not evaluated	53 to 63
Specificity	Not evaluated	29 to 75

REFERENCES

Laslett M. Evidence-based diagnosis and treatment of the painful sacroiliac joint. *J Man Manip Ther.* 2008;16(3):142-152.

Laslett M, Aprill CN, McDonald B, Young SB. Diagnosis of sacroiliac joint pain: validity of individual provocation tests and composites of tests. *Man Ther.* 2005;10(3):207-218.

Laslett M, Williams M. The reliability of selected pain provocation tests for sacroiliac joint pathology. *Spine (Phila Pa 1976).* 1994;19(11):1243-1249.

Levin U, Nilsson-Wikmar L, Stenström CH, Lundeberg T. Reproducibility of manual pressure force on provocation of the sacroiliac joint. *Physiother Res Int.* 1998;3(1):1-14.

Stuber KJ. Specificity, sensitivity, and predictive values of clinical tests of the sacroiliac joint: a systematic review of the literature. *J Can Chiropr Assoc.* 2007;51(1):30-41.

Szadek KM, van der Wurff P, van Tulder MW, Zuurmond WW, Perez RS. Diagnostic validity of criteria for sacroiliac joint pain: a systematic review. *J Pain.* 2009;10(4):354-368.

van der Wurff P, Hagmeijer RH, Meyne W. Clinical tests of the sacroiliac joint. A systematic methodological review. Part 1: reliability. *Man Ther.* 2000;5(1):30-36.

van der Wurff P, Meyne W, Hagmeijer RH. Clinical tests of the sacroiliac joint. *Man Ther.* 2000;5(2):89-96.

SACRAL SPINE

Squish Test

Test Positioning

The subject lies supine on the table while the examiner places a hand on each of the iliac crests and the anterior superior iliac spines of the subject (Figure SS8-4).

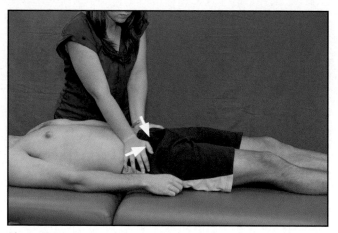

Figure SS8-4.

Action

The examiner compresses downward and inward at a 45-degree angle along the iliac crest and anterior superior iliac spine bilaterally.

Positive Finding

Subjective complaints of pain are noted as positive findings and may be found anteriorly or posteriorly.

Special Considerations/Comments

This test assesses the stability of the posterior SI ligaments but also directly applies compressive forces to the anterior SI joint. Thus, the location of pain should be noted and correlated with any additional findings.

YEOMAN'S TEST

TEST POSITIONING

The subject lies prone on the table.

ACTION

The examiner passively flexes the subject's knee to 90 degrees while simultaneously extending the ipsilateral hip (Figure SS8-5A).

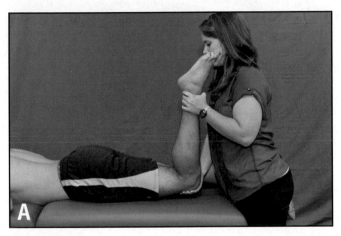

Figure SS8-5A.

POSITIVE FINDING

A reporting of pain during this test is considered to be a positive sign. Pain in the SI joint may be related to anterior SI ligament pathology. Pain in the anterior thigh region may be related to hip flexor musculature tightness or femoral nerve tension.

SPECIAL CONSIDERATIONS/COMMENTS

The examiner should pay attention to the position of the subject's trunk because trunk rotation may be used to compensate for positions of discomfort. Compensatory movement such as trunk rotation may result in a false-negative test finding (Figure SS8-5B).

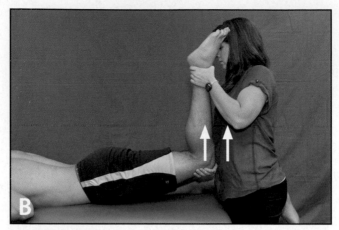

Figure SS8-5B.

REFERENCE

Walsh MJ. Evaluation of orthopedic testing of the low back for nonspecific lower back pain. *J Manipulative Physiol Ther.* 1998;21(4):232-236.

Gaenslen's Test

Test Positioning

The subject lies on the side of the uninvolved leg (lower leg). With the involved leg (upper leg) in slight hyperextension, the subject then flexes the hip and knee of the uninvolved side toward the chest.

Action

The examiner stabilizes the subject's pelvis and further extends the subject's involved leg (Figure SS8-6).

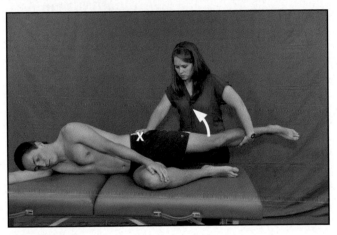

Figure SS8-6.

Positive Finding

Pain in the SI region is considered a positive finding and may be associated with SI joint dysfunction.

Special Considerations/Comments

The subject may report pain in the hip or anterior thigh region. This may be related to hip joint pathology, anterior thigh musculature tension, or L4 nerve root tension. This test can be performed with the subject in a supine position; however, the examiner should be cautious of a false-negative test due to the inability of obtaining enough involved leg hip extension.

EVIDENCE

	van der Wurff et al (2000)	Szadek et al (2009)
Study design	Systematic review	Systematic review
Conditions evaluated	SI joint pain	SI joint pain
Study number	2	3
Reliability	Kappa = .61 to .72	Not evaluated
Sensitivity	Not evaluated	50 to 71
Specificity	Not evaluated	26 to 79

REFERENCES

Laslett M. Evidence-based diagnosis and treatment of the painful sacro-iliac joint. *J Man Manip Ther.* 2008;16(3):142-152.

Laslett M, Aprill CN, McDonald B, Young SB. Diagnosis of sacroiliac joint pain: validity of individual provocation tests and composites of tests. *Man Ther.* 2005;10(3):207-218.

Laslett M, Williams M. The reliability of selected pain provocation tests for sacroiliac joint pathology. *Spine (Phila Pa 1976).* 1994;19(11):1243-1249.

Stuber KJ. Specificity, sensitivity, and predictive values of clinical tests of the sacroiliac joint: a systematic review of the literature. *J Can Chiropr Assoc.* 2007;51(1):30-41.

Szadek KM, van der Wurff P, van Tulder MW, Zuurmond WW, Perez RS. Diagnostic validity of criteria for sacroiliac joint pain: a systematic review. *J Pain.* 2009;10(4):354-368.

van der Wurff P, Hagmeijer RH, Meyne W. Clinical tests of the sacroiliac joint. A systematic methodological review. Part 1: reliability. *Man Ther.* 2000;5(1):30-36.

van der Wurff P, Meyne W, Hagmeijer RH. Clinical tests of the sacroiliac joint. *Man Ther.* 2000;5(2):89-96.

PATRICK OR FABER TEST

TEST POSITIONING

The subject lies supine on the table.

ACTION

The subject flexes, abducts, and externally rotates the involved leg until the foot rests on the top of the knee of the noninvolved lower extremity (Figure SS8-7A). The examiner then slowly abducts the involved lower extremity, bringing the knee closer toward the table (Figure SS8-7B).

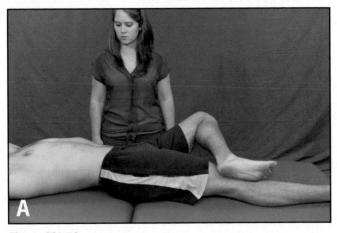

Figure SS8-7A.

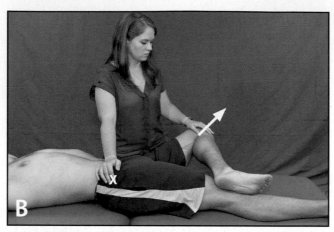

Figure SS8-7B.

POSITIVE FINDING

A positive finding is revealed when the involved lower extremity does not abduct below the level of the noninvolved lower extremity. This may be indicative of iliopsoas, SI, or even hip joint abnormalities.

SPECIAL CONSIDERATIONS/COMMENTS

FABER is an acronym for the initial positioning of the subject (flexion = F, abduction = AB, external rotation = ER).

EVIDENCE

	van der Wurff et al (2000)	Szadek et al (2009)
Study design	Systematic review	Systematic review
Conditions evaluated	SI joint pain	SI joint pain
Study number	3	3
Reliability	Kappa = .38 to .62	Not evaluated
Sensitivity	Not evaluated	63 to 100
Specificity	Not evaluated	16 to 77

REFERENCES

Brolinson PG, Maccoux DA, Gunter MJ. Groin pain—football. *Med Sci Sports Exerc.* 1997;29(5):30.

Cibulka MT, Delitto A. A comparison of two different methods to treat hip pain in runners. *J Orthop Sports Phys Ther.* 1993;17(4):172-176.

Cliborne AV, Wainner RS, Rhon DI, et al. Clinical hip tests and a functional squat test in patients with knee osteoarthritis: reliability, prevalence of positive test findings, and short-term response to hip mobilization. *J Orthop Sports Phys Ther.* 2004;34(11):676-685.

Mitchell B, McCrory P, Brukner P, O'Donnell J, Colson E, Howells R. Hip joint pathology: clinical presentation and correlation between magnetic resonance arthrography, ultrasound, and arthroscopic findings in 25 consecutive cases. *Clin J Sport Med.* 2003;13(3):152-156.

Ross MD, Nordeen MH, Barido M. Test-retest reliability of Patrick's hip range of motion test in healthy college-aged men. *J Strength Cond Res.* 2003;17(1):156-161.

Strender LE, Sjöblom A, Sundell K, Ludwig R, Taube A. Interexaminer reliability in physical examination of patients with low back pain. *Spine (Phila Pa 1976).* 1997;22(7):814-820.

Szadek KM, van der Wurff P, van Tulder MW, Zuurmond WW, Perez RS. Diagnostic validity of criteria for sacroiliac joint pain: a systematic review. *J Pain.* 2009;10(4):354-368.

van der Wurff P, Hagmeijer RH, Meyne W. Clinical tests of the sacroiliac joint. A systematic methodological review. Part 1: Reliability. *Man Ther.* 2000;5(1):30-36.

LONG-SITTING TEST

TEST POSITIONING

The subject lies supine with both hips and knees extended, and the examiner stands with the thumbs on the subject's medial malleoli (Figure SS8-8A).

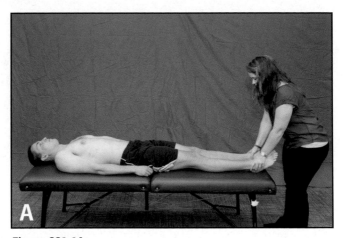

Figure SS8-8A.

ACTION

The examiner passively flexes both knees and hips (Figure SS8-8B) and then fully extends and compares the position of the medial malleoli relative to each other (Figure SS8-8C). The subject then slowly assumes the long-sitting position, and the malleolar position is re-assessed (Figures SS8-8D and SS8-8E).

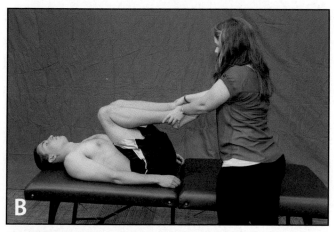

Figure SS8-8B.

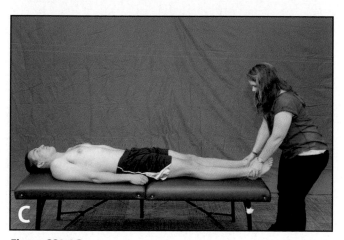

Figure SS8-8C.

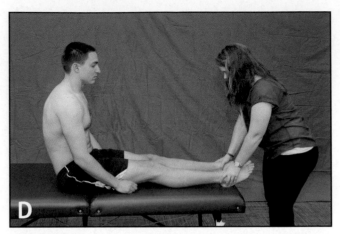

Figure SS8-8D.

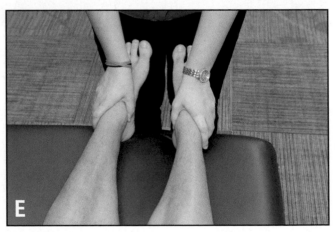

Figure SS8-8E.

POSITIVE FINDING

A leg that appears longer in the supine position but shorter in the long-sitting position is indicative of an ipsilateral anteriorly rotated ilium. Conversely, a leg that appears shorter in the supine position but longer in the long-sitting position is indicative of an ipsilateral posteriorly rotated ilium.

SPECIAL CONSIDERATIONS/COMMENTS

Marking the reference point of measurement on the malleoli with a pen may increase the reliability when comparing positions of leg length.

EVIDENCE

	van der Wurff et al (2000)
Study design	Systematic review
Conditions evaluated	SI joint mobility
Study number	1
Reliability	% agreement = 40
Sensitivity	Not evaluated
Specificity	Not evaluated

REFERENCES

Bemis T, Daniel M. Validation of the long-sitting test on subjects with ilio-sacral dysfunction. *J Orthop Sports Phys Ther.* 1987;8(7):336-345.

van der Wurff P, Hagmeijer RH, Meyne W. Clinical tests of the sacroiliac joint. A systematic methodological review. Part 1: reliability. *Man Ther.* 2000;5(1):30-36.

SACRAL SPINE

Please see videos on the accompanying website at
www.healio.com/books/specialtestsvideos

Section
9

Hip

Guide to Figures

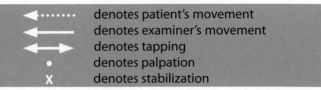

◄······· denotes patient's movement
◄———— denotes examiner's movement
◄———► denotes tapping
• denotes palpation
x denotes stabilization

Konin JG, Lebsack D, Snyder Valier AR, Isear JA Jr.
Special Tests for Orthopedic Examination, Fourth Edition (pp 237-268).
© 2016 SLACK Incorporated.

HIP SCOURING/QUADRANT TEST

TEST POSITIONING

The subject lies supine. The examiner stands on the involved side and passively flexes and adducts the subject's hip. The subject's knee is also placed in full flexion (Figure H9-1A).

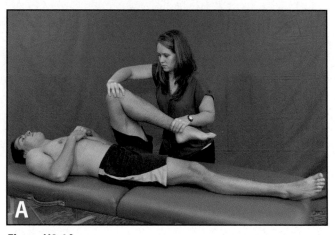

Figure H9-1A.

ACTION

The examiner applies downward pressure along the shaft of the femur while simultaneously adducting and externally rotating the hip (Figure H9-1B). The examiner then adducts and internally rotates the hip while maintaining downward pressure (Figure H9-1C). This movement is repeated 2 to 3 times while the examiner notes any unusual movement (ie, catching, grinding) or subject apprehension.

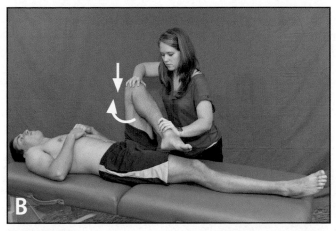

Figure H9-1B.

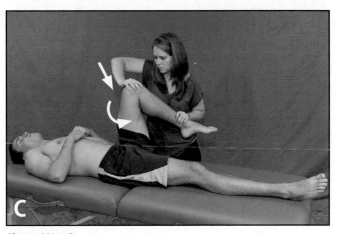

Figure H9-1C.

POSITIVE FINDING

Pain or apprehension is indicative of hip joint pathology, such as arthritis, osteochondral defects, avascular necrosis, or acetabular labrum defects.

SPECIAL CONSIDERATIONS/COMMENTS

This test is not very specific for identifying structural damage and should be used with caution to avoid causing further pain and/or tissue damage. Imaging tests are helpful tools to use in follow-up of a positive hip scour test accompanied by unexplained hip joint and/or radiating leg pain.

EVIDENCE

	Reiman et al (2013)
Study design	Systematic review
Conditions evaluated	Hip pathologies
Study number	1
Reliability	Not evaluated
Sensitivity	50
Specificity	29

REFERENCES

Margo K, Drezner J, Motzkin D. Evaluation and management of hip pain: an algorithmic approach. *J Fam Prac.* 2003;52(8):607-617.

Mitchell B, McCrory P, Brukner P, O'Donnell J, Colson E, Howells R. Hip joint pathology: clinical presentation and correlation between magnetic resonance arthrography, ultrasound, and arthroscopic findings in 25 consecutive cases. *Clin J Sport Med.* 2003;13(3):152-156.

Narvani AA, Tsiridis E, Kendall S, Chaudhuri R, Thomas P. A preliminary report on prevalence of acetabular labrum tears in sports patients with groin pain. *Knee Surg Sports Traumatol Arthrosc.* 2003;11(6):403-408.

Reiman MP, Goode AP, Hegedus EJ, Cook CE, Wright AA. Diagnostic accuracy of clinical tests of the hip: a systematic review with meta-analysis. *Br J Sports Med.* 2013;47(14):893-902.

HIP

CRAIG'S TEST

TEST POSITIONING

The subject lies prone with the affected leg's knee flexed to 90 degrees. The examiner stands on the involved side and palpates the greater trochanter (Figure H9-2A).

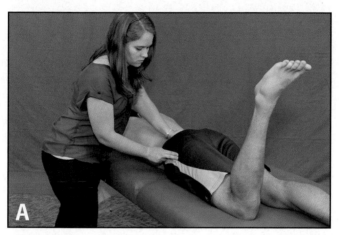

Figure H9-2A.

ACTION

The examiner then passively internally and externally rotates the femur until the greater trochanter is parallel with the examining table (Figure H9-2B). At this point, the subject is asked to hold the hip in this position while the examiner measures the angle between the long axis of the lower leg and the perpendicular axis to the table with a goniometer (Figure H9-2C).

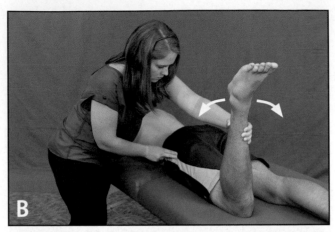

Figure H9-2B. Note: Internal/external rotation of the hip until the greater trochanter is parallel with the table.

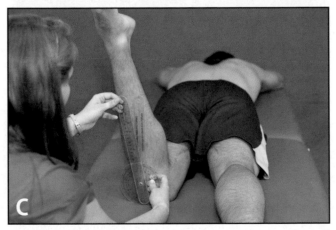

Figure H9-2C. Note: Femoral anteversion > 15 degrees; femoral retroversion < 8 degrees.

POSITIVE FINDING

If the measured angle is greater than 15 degrees, femoral anteversion is indicated. If the measured angle is less than 8 degrees, femoral retroversion is indicated. Increased femoral anteversion leads to toeing-in and squinting patellae. Femoral retroversion leads to a toeing-out position. Both of these may lead to lower extremity malalignment and subsequent pathologies.

SPECIAL CONSIDERATIONS/COMMENTS

A second examiner may be useful to hold the subject's hip and leg in the designated position while the first examiner measures the angle. This test is also known as the Ryder Method for measuring femoral anteversion and retroversion.

REFERENCES

Dunn DM. Anteversion of the neck of the femur; a method of measurement. *J Bone Joint Surg Br.* 1952;34(2):181-186.

Ryder CT, Crane L. Measuring femoral anteversion; the problem and a method. *J Bone Joint Surg Am.* 1953;35(2):321-328.

Hip

90-90 STRAIGHT LEG RAISE TEST

TEST POSITIONING

Test subject lies supine, stabilizing both hips at 90 degrees of flexion with both hands. The knees are bent in a relaxed position. The examiner stands next to the subject (Figure H9-3A).

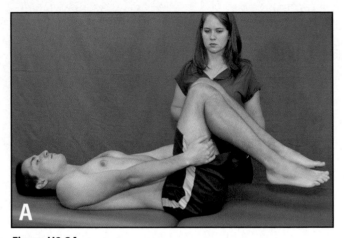

Figure H9-3A.

ACTION

The subject is instructed to actively extend one knee at a time as much as possible (Figure H9-3B). The test is performed bilaterally.

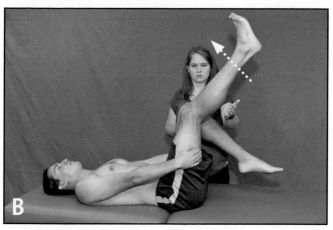

Figure H9-3B.

POSITIVE FINDING

If the knee is flexed greater than 20 degrees, the hamstrings are considered tight.

SPECIAL CONSIDERATIONS/COMMENTS

When assessing this test, care should always be taken to be consistent with the position of the pelvis so that testing measures can be repeated with reliability.

REFERENCES

Cameron DM, Bohannon RW. Relationship between active knee extension and active straight leg raise test measurements. *J Orthop Sports Phys Ther.* 1993;17(5):257-260.

Draper DO, Castro JL, Feland B, Schulthies S, Eggett D. Shortwave diathermy and prolonged stretching increase hamstring flexibility more than prolonged stretching alone. *J Orthop Sports Phys Ther.* 2004;34(1):13-20.

Gabbe BJ, Bennell KL, Wajswelner H, Finch CF. Reliability of common lower extremity musculoskeletal screening tests. *Phys Ther Sport.* 2004;5(2):90-97.

Gajdosik RL, Rieck MA, Sullivan DK, Wightman SE. Comparison of four clinical tests for assessing hamstring muscle length. *J Orthop Sports Phys Ther.* 1993;18(5):614-618.

Tafazzoli F, Lamontagne M. Mechanical behaviour of hamstring muscles in low-back pain patients and control subjects. *Clin Biomech (Bristol, Avon).* 1996;11(1):16-24.

PATRICK OR FABER TEST

TEST POSITIONING

The subject lies supine on the table.

ACTION

The subject flexes, abducts, and externally rotates the involved leg until the foot rests on the top of the knee of the noninvolved lower extremity (Figure H9-4A). The examiner then slowly abducts the involved lower extremity, bringing the knee closer toward the table (Figure H9-4B).

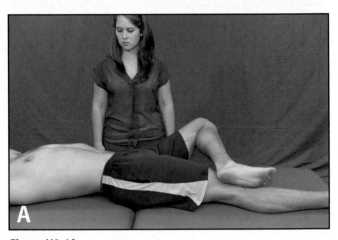

Figure H9-4A.

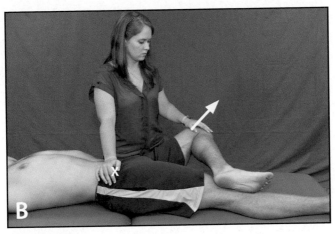

Figure H9-4B.

POSITIVE FINDING

A positive finding is revealed when the involved lower extremity does not abduct below the level of the noninvolved lower extremity. This may be indicative of iliopsoas, sacroiliac, or even hip joint abnormalities.

SPECIAL CONSIDERATIONS/COMMENTS

FABER is an acronym for the initial positioning of the subject (flexion = F, abduction = AB, external rotation = ER).

EVIDENCE

	Reiman et al (2013)
Study design	Systematic review
Conditions evaluated	Hip pathologies
Study number	4
Reliability	Not evaluated
Sensitivity	42 to 81
Specificity	18 to 75

Hip

REFERENCES

Brolinson PG, Maccoux DA, Gunter MJ. Groin pain—football. *Med Sci Sports Exerc.* 1997;29(5):30.

Cibulka MT, Delitto A. A comparison of two different methods to treat hip pain in runners. *J Orthop Sports Phys Ther.* 1993;17(4):172-176.

Cliborne AV, Wainner RS, Rhon DI, et al. Clinical hip tests and a functional squat test in patients with knee osteoarthritis: reliability, prevalence of positive test findings, and short-term response to hip mobilization. *J Orthop Sports Phys Ther.* 2004;34(11):676-685.

Mitchell B, McCrory P, Brukner P, O'Donnell J, Colson E, Howells R. Hip joint pathology: clinical presentation and correlation between magnetic resonance arthrography, ultrasound, and arthroscopic findings in 25 consecutive cases. *Clin J Sport Med.* 2003;13(3):152-156.

Reiman MP, Goode AP, Hegedus EJ, Cook CE, Wright AA. Diagnostic accuracy of clinical tests of the hip: a systematic review with meta-analysis. *Br J Sports Med.* 2013;47(14):893-902.

Ross MD, Nordeen MH, Barido M. Test-retest reliability of Patrick's hip range of motion test in healthy college-aged men. *J Strength Cond Res.* 2003;17(1):156-161.

Strender LE, Sjöblom A, Sundell K, Ludwig R, Taube A. Interexaminer reliability in physical examination of patients with low back pain. *Spine (Phila Pa 1976).* 1997;22(7):814-820.

Hip

TRENDELENBURG'S TEST

TEST POSITIONING

The subject stands on one lower extremity (Figure H9-5A).

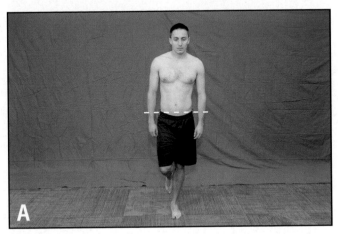

Figure H9-5A.

ACTION

The subject remains in this position for approximately 10 seconds and then switches extremities.

POSITIVE FINDING

A positive finding is seen when the pelvis on the unsupported side drops noticeably lower than the pelvis on the supported side (Figure H9-5B). This indicates a weakness of the gluteus medius muscle on the supported side. Figures H9-5C and H9-5D show the posterior view.

HIP

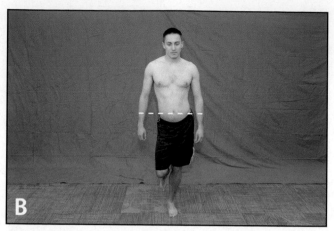

Figure H9-5B.

SPECIAL CONSIDERATIONS/COMMENTS

With a negative test, the gluteus medius on the supported side will perform a reverse action because the supported femur is stabilized. This will allow for the unsupported pelvis to remain level with the supported pelvis. With a weak gluteus medius on the supported side, the unsupported pelvis drops as the muscle fatigues. This test may also indicate an unstable hip on the supported side.

EVIDENCE

	Reiman et al (2013)
Study design	Meta-analysis
Conditions evaluated	Gluteal tendinopathy
Study number	3
Sample size	78
Reliability	Not evaluated
Sensitivity	61
Specificity	92

Hip

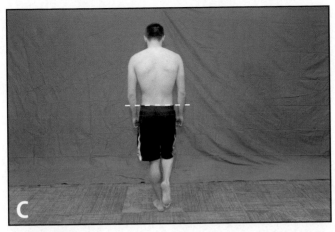

Figure H9-5C.

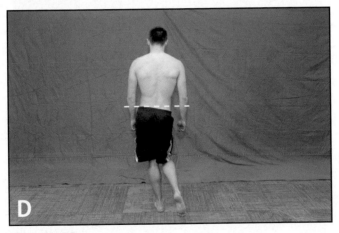

Figure H9-5D.

References

Asayama I, Naito M, Fujisawa M, Kambe T. Relationship between radiographic measurements of reconstructed hip joint position and the Trendelenburg sign. *J Arthroplasty.* 2002;17(6):747-751.

Bird PA, Oakley SP, Shnier R, Kirkham BW. Prospective evaluation of magnetic resonance imaging and physical examination findings in patients with greater trochanteric pain syndrome. *Arthritis Rheum.* 2001;44(9):2138-2145.

Hardcastle P, Nade S. The significance of the Trendelenburg test. *J Bone Joint Surg Br.* 1985;67(5):741-746.

Reiman MP, Goode AP, Hegedus EJ, Cook CE, Wright AA. Diagnostic accuracy of clinical tests of the hip: a systematic review with meta-analysis. *Br J Sports Med.* 2013;47(14):893-902.

Trendelenburg F. Trendelenburg's test: 1895. *Clin Orthop Relat Res.* 1998;(355):3-7.

Vasudevan PN, Vaidyalingam KV, Nair PB. Can Trendelenburg's sign be positive if the hip is normal? *J Bone Joint Surg Br.* 1997;79(3):462-466.

Youdas JW, Madson TJ, Hollman JH. Usefulness of the Trendelenburg test for identification of patients with hip joint osteoarthritis. *Physiother Theory Pract.* 26(3):184-194.

Hip

Ober's Test

Test Positioning

The subject lies on the side with the hips and knees extended so that the test leg is superior to the nontest leg. The examiner stands behind the subject with the proximal hand stabilizing the pelvis and the distal hand supporting the lower leg (Figure H9-6A). The knee of the test leg is flexed to 90 degrees.

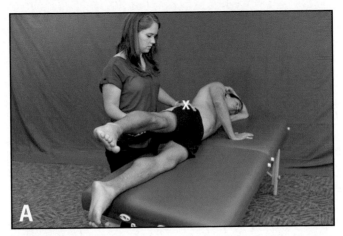

Figure H9-6A.

HIP

Action

The knee of the test leg is flexed to 90 degrees. With the pelvis stabilized to prevent rolling, abduct and extend the test hip to position the iliotibial band behind the greater trochanter (Figure H9-6B). Then allow the leg to slowly lower (adduct).

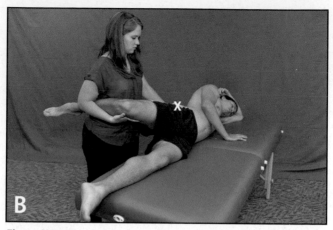

Figure H9-6B.

POSITIVE FINDING

The inability of the leg to adduct and touch the table is indicative of iliotibial band tightness (particularly the tensor fasciae latae). The leg will react like a "springboard" because the leg remains abducted in mid-air (Figure H9-6C).

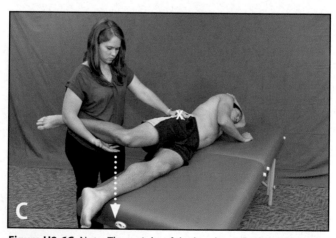

Figure H9-6C. Note: The weight of the leg drops the leg toward the table.

Hip

SPECIAL CONSIDERATIONS/COMMENTS

It is important to apply a downward force on the ilium near the crest while allowing the leg to adduct. This will prevent lateral tilting (ie, inferior movement) of the pelvis on the side of the test leg, which could give a false-negative result. Additionally, it is important to ensure complete relaxation of the hip abductor muscles. It may be helpful to have the subject actively adduct the test leg into the support hand and then relax to inhibit hip abductor muscle guarding. This test was originally described by Ober to be performed with the knee flexed to 90 degrees. However, it has been modified (ie, Modified Ober's Test) because it is believed that a greater stretch is placed on the iliotibial band when the knee is in an extended position. Furthermore, performing this test with the knee in flexion places greater tension on the femoral nerve, requiring the examiner to be cognizant of associated neurological complaints.

EVIDENCE

	Reese and Bandy (2003)	Ferber et al (2010)
Study design	Reliability	Cross-sectional
Conditions evaluated	Iliotibial band tightness	Iliotibial band tightness
Sample size	61	300
Reliability	Intrarater reliability = .90	Interrater agreement = 97.6%
Sensitivity	Not evaluated	Not evaluated
Specificity	Not evaluated	Not evaluated

REFERENCES

Ferber R, Kendall KD, McElroy L. Normative and critical criteria for iliotibial band and iliopsoas muscle flexibility. *J Athl Train.* 2010;45(4):344-348.

Fredericson M, White JJ, Macmahon JM, Andriachi TP. Quantitative analysis of the relative effectiveness of 3 iliotibial band stretches. *Arch Phys Med Rehabil.* 2002;83(5):589-592.

Hip

Gajdosik RL, Sandler MM, Marr HL. Influence of knee positions and gender on the Ober test for length of the iliotibial band. *Clin Biomech (Bristol, Avon).* 2003;18(1):77-79.

Gautam VK, Anand S. A new test for estimating iliotibial band contracture. *J Bone Joint Surg Br.* 1998;80(3):474-475.

Margo K, Drezner J, Motzkin D. Evaluation and management of hip pain: an algorithmic approach. *J Fam Prac.* 2003;52(8):607-617.

Melchione WE, Sullivan MS. Reliability of measurements obtained by use of an instrument designed to indirectly measure iliotibial band length. *J Orthop Sports Phys Ther.* 1993;18(3):511-515.

Ober FB. The role of the iliotibial and fascia lata as a factor in the causation of low-back disabilities and sciatica. *J Bone Joint Surg.* 1936;18:105.

Reese NB, Bandy WD. Use of an inclinometer to measure flexibility of the iliotibial band using the Ober test and the modified Ober test: differences in magnitude and reliability of measurements. *J Orthop Sports Phys Ther.* 2003;33(6):326-330.

Winslow J, Yoder E. Patellofemoral pain in female ballet dancers: correlation with iliotibial band tightness and tibial external rotation. *J Orthop Sports Phys Ther.* 1995;22(1):18-21.

Hip

Piriformis Test

TEST POSITIONING

The subject lies on the nontest side with the test leg in 60 degrees of hip flexion and relaxed knee flexion. The examiner stands with the proximal hand on the subject's pelvis (laterally) and the distal hand on the subject's knee (laterally) (Figure H9-7).

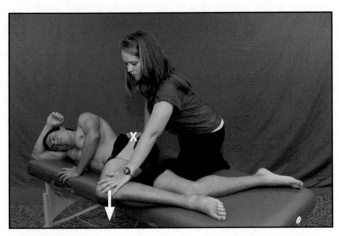

Figure H9-7.

ACTION

With the subject's pelvis stabilized, apply an adduction (downward) force on the subject's knee.

POSITIVE FINDING

Tightness or pain in the hip and buttock areas is indicative of piriformis tightness. Pain in the buttock and posterior thigh is indicative of sciatic nerve impingement secondary to piriformis tightness.

SPECIAL CONSIDERATIONS/COMMENTS

This test may also be performed with the subject supine. It is important for the examiner to differentiate between subjective complaints of pain that may be reported in the hip area but are not actually associated with a tight piriformis muscle.

REFERENCES

Broadhurst NA, Simmons DN, Bond MJ. Piriformis syndrome: correlation of muscle morphology with symptoms and signs. *Arch Phys Med Rehabil.* 2004;85(12):2036-2039.

Fishman LM, Dombi GW, Michaelsen C, et al. Piriformis syndrome: diagnosis, treatment, and outcome—a 10-year study. *Arch Phys Med Rehabil.* 2002;83(5):295-301.

Fishman LM, Schaefer MP. The Piriformis syndrome is underdiagnosed. *Muscle Nerve.* 2003;28(5):646-649.

Stewart JD. The Piriformis syndrome is overdiagnosed. *Muscle Nerve.* 2003;28(5):644-646.

THOMAS TEST

TEST POSITIONING

The subject lies supine with both knees fully flexed against the chest and the buttocks near the table edge. The examiner stands with one hand on the subject's lumbar spine or iliac crest to monitor lumbar lordosis or pelvic tilt, respectively (Figure H9-8A).

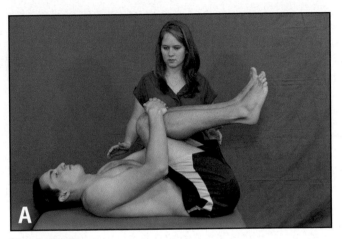

Figure H9-8A.

ACTION

The subject slowly lowers the test leg until the leg is fully relaxed or until either anterior pelvic tilting or an increase in lumbar lordosis occurs (Figure H9-8B).

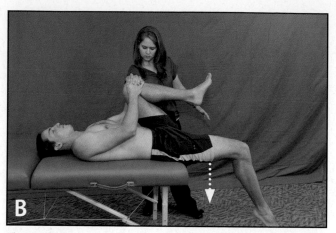

Figure H9-8B.

POSITIVE FINDING

A lack of hip extension with knee flexion greater than 45 degrees is indicative of iliopsoas muscle tightness. Full hip extension with knee flexion less than 45 degrees is indicative of rectus femoris muscle tightness. A lack of hip extension with knee flexion less than 45 degrees is indicative of iliopsoas and rectus femoris muscle tightness. Hip external rotation during any of the previous scenarios is indicative of iliotibial band tightness.

SPECIAL CONSIDERATIONS/COMMENTS

Increases in anterior pelvic tilt and lumbar lordosis must be eliminated to prevent false-negative findings. To further confirm this assessment, the examiner can simply apply pressure on the lower leg in an effort to lower it back to the table. A return of lumbar lordosis will indicate a positive finding.

HIP

EVIDENCE

	Reiman et al (2013)
Study design	Systematic review
Conditions evaluated	Hip pathology
Study number	1
Reliability	Not evaluated
Sensitivity	89
Specificity	92

REFERENCES

Barlett MD, Wolf LS, Shurtleff DB, Staheli LT. Hip flexion contractures: a comparison of measurement methods. *Arch Phys Med Rehabil.* 1985;66(9):620-625.

Eland DC, Singleton TN, Conaster RR, et al. The "iliacus test": new information for the evaluation of hip extension dysfunction. *J Am Osteopath Assoc.* 2002;102(3):130-142.

Gabbe BJ, Bennell KL, Wajswelner H, Finch CF. Reliability of common lower extremity musculoskeletal screening tests. *Phys Ther Sport.* 2004;5(2):90-97.

Harvey D. Assessment of the flexibility of elite athletes using the modified Thomas test. *Br J Sports Med.* 1998;32(1)68-70.

Harvey DM. Flexibility of elite athletes using the modified Thomas test. *Med Sci Sport Exerc.* 1997;29(5):271.

Koyama H, Murakami K, Suzuki T, Suzaki K. Phenol block for hip flexor muscle spasticity under ultrasonic monitoring. *Arch Phys Med Rehabil.* 1992;73(11):1040-1043.

Lee LW, Kerrigan D. Casey MD, Croce UD. Dynamic implications of hip flexion contractures. *Am J Phys Med Rehabil.* 1997;76(6):502-508.

Margo K, Drezner J, Motzkin D. Evaluation and management of hip pain: an algorithmic approach. *J Fam Pract.* 2003;52(8):607-617.

Narvani AA, Tsiridis E, Kendall S, Chaudhuri R, Thomas P. A preliminary report on prevalence of acetabular labrum tears in sports patients with groin pain. *Knee Surg Sports Traumatol Arthrosc.* 2003;11(6):403-408.

Reiman MP, Goode AP, Hegedus EJ, Cook CE, Wright AA. Diagnostic accuracy of clinical tests of the hip: a systematic review with meta-analysis. *Br J Sports Med.* 2013;47(14):893-902.

Schache AG, Blanch PD, Murphy AT. Relation of anterior pelvic tilt during running to clinical and kinematic measures of hip extension. *Br J Sports Med.* 2000;34(4):279-283.

Tyler T, Zook L, Brittis D, Gleim G. A new pelvic tilt detection device: roentgenographic validation and application to assessment of hip motion in professional ice hockey players. *J Orthop Sports Phys Ther.* 1996;24(5):303-308.

Winters MV, Blake CG, Trost JS, et al. Passive versus active stretching of hip flexor muscles in subjects with limited hip extension: a randomized clinical trial. *Phys Ther.* 2004;84(9):800-807.

Young W, Clothier P, Otago L, Bruce L, Liddell D. Acute effects of static stretching on hip flexor and quadriceps flexibility, range of motion and foot speed in kicking a football. *J Sci Med Sport.* 2004;7(1):23-31.

ELY'S TEST

TEST POSITIONING

The subject lies prone. The examiner stands on one side of the table next to the subject's leg, placing one hand over the ipsilateral pelvic region.

ACTION

The examiner passively flexes the subject's knee and notes the reaction at the hip joint. This test is repeated on the other side for comparison (Figure H9-9A).

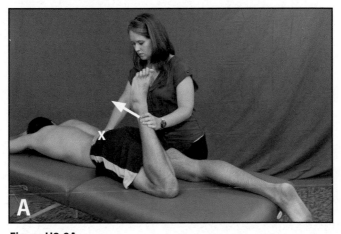

Figure H9-9A.

POSITIVE FINDING

If the hip also flexes when the knee is flexed, a tight rectus femoris is indicated (Figure H9-9B).

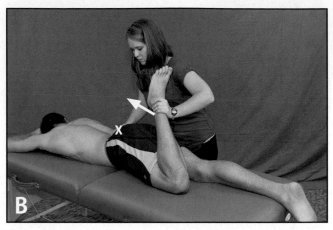

Figure H9-9B.

SPECIAL CONSIDERATIONS/COMMENTS

This test may be uncomfortable when performed on a subject who has pelvic or sacroiliac dysfunction because of the prone positioning.

EVIDENCE

	Peeler and Anderson (2008)
Study design	Reliability
Conditions evaluated	Rectus femoris flexibility
Sample size	54
Reliability	Intrarater: Kappa = .46 to .62
	Interrater: Kappa = .42 to .52
Sensitivity	Not evaluated
Specificity	Not evaluated

REFERENCES

Duncan JA. Medical care of young persons in industry. *Public Health.* 1955;68(9):136-139.

Kay RM, Rethlefsen SA, Kelly JP, Wren TAL. Predictive value of the Duncan-Ely test in distal rectus femoris transfer. *J Pediatr Orthop.* 2004;24(1):59-62.

Marks MC, Alexander J, Sutherland DH, Chambers HG. Clinical utility of the Duncan-Ely test for rectus femoris dysfunction during the swing phase of gait. *Dev Med Child Neurol.* 2003;45(11):763-768.

Peeler J, Anderson JE. Reliability of the Ely's test for assessing rectus femoris muscle flexibility and joint range of motion. *J Orthop Res.* 2008;26(6):793-799.

FEMORAL NERVE TRACTION TEST

TEST POSITIONING

The subject lies on the uninvolved side with the hip and knee slightly flexed. The examiner places one hand on the lateral aspect of the subject's involved pelvis while the other hand supports the leg below the knee.

ACTION

The subject slightly flexes the head while the examiner completely extends the subject's knee and extends the hip approximately 15 degrees (Figure H9-10A). The examiner then flexes the subject's knee (Figure H9-10B).

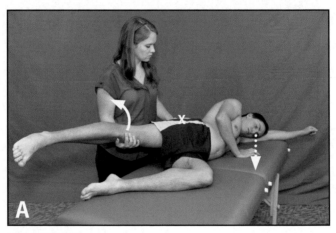

Figure H9-10A.

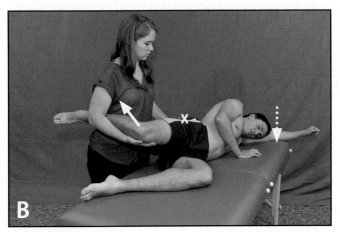

Figure H9-10B.

POSITIVE FINDING

The motion of hip extension and knee flexion places the femoral nerve on stretch. Subjective complaints of pain along the anterior thigh region may indicate decreased mobilization of the femoral nerve.

SPECIAL CONSIDERATIONS/COMMENTS

The subject's spine should be in a neutral position. The location of subjectively reported pain should be carefully considered so that the examiner can differentiate between nerve roots.

Hip

REFERENCES

Christodoulides AN. Ipsilateral sciatica on femoral nerve stretch test is pathognomonic of an L4/5 disk protrusion. *J Bone Joint Surg Br.* 1989;71(1):88-89.

Dyck P. The femoral nerve traction test with lumbar disk protrusions. *Surg Neurol.* 1976;3:163-166.

Nadler SF, Malanga GA, Stitik TP, Keswani R, Foye PM. The crossed femoral nerve stretch test to improve diagnostic sensitivity for the high lumbar radiculopathy: 2 case reports. *Arch Phys Med Rehab.* 2001;82(4):522-523.

HIP

Please see videos on the accompanying website at
www.healio.com/books/specialtestsvideos

Section

10

Knee

Guide to Figures

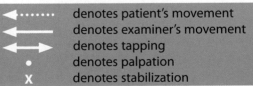

◄······· denotes patient's movement
◄───── denotes examiner's movement
◄────► denotes tapping
  •   denotes palpation
  x   denotes stabilization

Konin JG, Lebsack D, Snyder Valier AR, Isear JA Jr.
Special Tests for Orthopedic Examination, Fourth Edition (pp 269-361).
© 2016 SLACK Incorporated.

PATELLA TENDON/PATELLA LIGAMENT LENGTH TEST

TEST POSITIONING

The subject lies supine on a table.

ACTION

The examiner measures the distance between the superior pole of the patella and the inferior pole of the patella (Figure K10-1A). The examiner then measures the distance between the inferior pole of the patella and the tibial tubercle (Figure K10-1B).

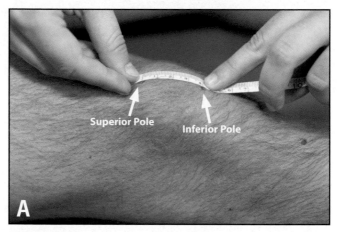

Figure K10-1A.

POSITIVE FINDING

A ratio is taken between the first and second measurements. A ratio greater than one indicates patella baja, whereas a ratio less than one indicates patella alta.

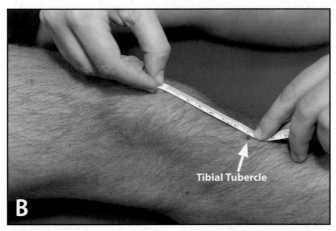

Figure K10-1B.

SPECIAL CONSIDERATIONS/COMMENTS

Patella alta may predispose one to increased instability of the patellofemoral joint, whereas patella baja may predispose one to increased patellofemoral compressive forces and related pathologies.

REFERENCES

Hirano A, Fukubayashi T, Ishii T, Ochiai N. Relationship between the patellar height and the disorder of the knee extensor mechanism in immature athletes. *J Pediatr Orthop.* 2001;21(4):541-544.

Kadakia NR, Ilahi OA. Interobserver variability of the Insall-Salvati ratio. *Orthopedics.* 2003;26(3):321-323; discussion 323-324.

Lin CF, Wu JJ, Chen TS, Huang TF. Comparison of the Insall-Salvati ratio of the patella in patients with and without an ACL tear. *Knee Surg Sports Traumatol Arthrosc.* 2004;13(1):8-11.

Neyret P, Robinson AH, Le Coultre B, Lapra C, Chambat P. Patellar tendon length—the factor in patellar instability? *Knee.* 2002;9(1):3-6.

Seil R, Müller B, Georg T, Kohn D, Rupp S. Reliability and interobserver variability in radiological patellar height ratios. *Knee Surg Sports Traumatol Arthrosc.* 2000;8(4):231-236.

Shabshin N, Schweitzer ME, Morrison WB, Parker L. MRI criteria for patella alta and baja. *Skeletal Radiol.* 2004;33(8):445-450.

PATELLAR APPREHENSION TEST

TEST POSITIONING

The subject lies supine with both knees fully extended. The examiner stands opposite the involved side and places both thumbs on the medial border of the patella being tested (Figure K10-2A).

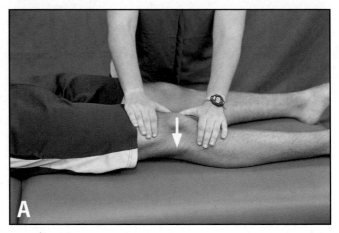

Figure K10-2A. Note: The examiner stands on the opposite side and passively glides the patella laterally.

ACTION

The subject must remain relaxed with no quadriceps contraction while the examiner gently pushes the patella laterally.

POSITIVE FINDING

If the subject is apprehensive to this movement or contracts the quadriceps muscle to protect against subluxation, the test is indicative of patellar subluxation or dislocation (possibly due to laxity of the medial retinaculum).

KNEE

Special Considerations/Comments

The action may be repeated with the knee flexed to 30 degrees (Figure K10-2B). The examiner must avoid excessive lateral patellar glide to prevent patellar dislocation. The patient's face can also be watched for a look of apprehension.

Figure K10-2B is also called Fairbanks Apprehension Test (knee is at 30 degrees of flexion).

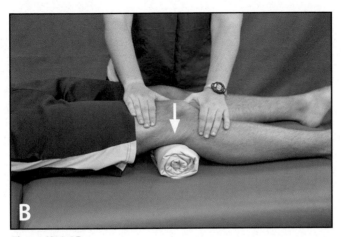

Figure K10-2B.

Evidence

	Cook et al (2012)
Study design	Systematic review
Conditions evaluated	Patellar femoral pain syndrome
Study number	3
Reliability	Not evaluated
Sensitivity	7 to 37
Specificity	70 to 92

REFERENCES

Cook C, Mabry L, Reiman MP, Hegedus EJ. Best tests/clinical findings for screening and diagnosis of patellofemoral pain syndrome: a systematic review. *Physiotherapy.* 2012;98(2):93-100.

Dimon JH III. Apprehension test for subluxation of the patella. *Clin Orthop Relat Res.* 1974;103:39.

Niskanen RO, Paavilainen PJ, Jaakkola M, Korkala OL. Poor correlation of clinical signs with patellar cartilaginous changes. *Arthroscopy.* 2001;17(3):307-310.

Tanner SM, Garth WP Jr, Soileau R, Lemons JE. A modified test for patellar instability: the biomechanical basis. *Clin J Sport Med.* 2003;13(6):327-338.

BALLOTABLE PATELLA OR PATELLA TAP TEST

TEST POSITIONING

The subject lies supine with both knees fully extended. The examiner stands with the proximal hand over the suprapatellar pouch and the distal hand (thumb or first 2 fingers) over the patella (Figure K10-3).

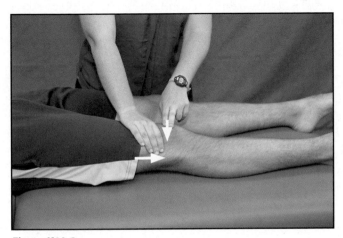

Figure K10-3.

ACTION

Compress the suprapatellar pouch with the proximal hand, then compress the patella into the femur.

POSITIVE FINDING

Downward movement of the patella followed by a rebound will give the appearance of a floating or ballotable patella and is indicative of moderate to severe joint effusion.

KNEE

SPECIAL CONSIDERATIONS/COMMENTS

If a ballotable patella is determined, the examiner should take girth measurements at the supra-, mid-, and infrapatellar regions and compare them bilaterally to more accurately assess the severity/degree of effusion. Additionally, the examiner must not mistake prepatellar bursitis as a joint effusion. The former will present as a "raw egg" over the patella, but no downward patellar movement will be present. Occasionally, concomitant joint effusion and prepatellar bursitis will be present and the examiner will therefore be challenged to make the proper assessment.

EVIDENCE

	Pookarnjanamorakot et al (2004)
Study design	Cross-sectional
Conditions evaluated	Meniscal injuries
Sample size	100
Reliability	Not evaluated
Sensitivity	32
Specificity	100

REFERENCES

Johnson MW. Acute knee effusions: a systematic approach to diagnosis. *Am Fam Physician.* 2000;61(8):2391-2400.

Pookarnjanamorakot C, Korsantirat T, Woratanarat P. Meniscal lesions in the anterior cruciate insufficient knee: the accuracy of clinical evaluation. *J Med Assoc Thai.* 2004;87(6):618-623.

SWEEP TEST (WIPE, BRUSH, BULGE, OR STROKE TEST)

TEST POSITIONING

The subject lies supine with the involved knee in full extension. The examiner places both hands on the medial aspect of the patella.

ACTION

The examiner attempts to "milk" or "sweep" any intracapsular swelling by applying pressure to the proximal (Figure K10-4A), distal (Figure K10-4B), and lateral (Figure K10-4C) aspects of the patella.

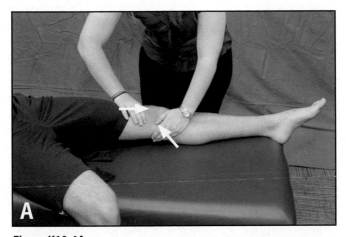

Figure K10-4A.

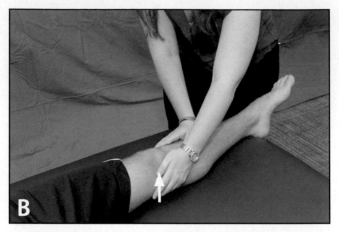

Figure K10-4B.

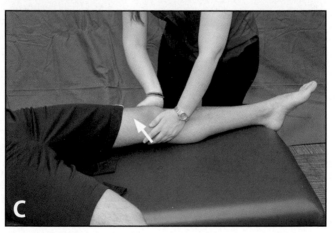

Figure K10-4C.

POSITIVE FINDING

Fluid that accumulates on the medial aspect of the patella is representative of intracapsular swelling.

SPECIAL CONSIDERATIONS/COMMENTS

Intracapsular swelling can be the result of damage to any internal capsular structure. The subject should maintain muscle relaxation during this test. This test is also referred to as the Wipe, Brush, Bulge, or Stroke Test.

REFERENCE

Stiell IG, Wells GA, Greenberg GH, et al. Interobserver agreement in the examination of patients with acute knee injury. *Ann Emerg Med.* 1996;27(1):136-137.

Q-ANGLE TEST

TEST POSITIONING

The subject lies supine with the hips and knees extended.

ACTION

Identify the anterior superior iliac spines, midpoint of the patella, and the tibial tubercle. Strike a line from the anterior superior iliac spines to the midpoint of the patella and from the tibial tubercle to the midpoint of the patella. Place a goniometer on the knee so that the axis is over the midpoint of the patella, the proximal arm is over the line to the anterior superior iliac spines, and the distal arm is over the line to the tibial tubercle. The resultant angle is the Q-angle (Figure K10-5).

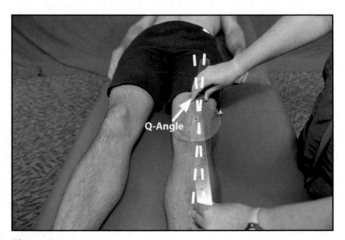

Figure K10-5.

POSITIVE FINDING

Q-angle norms with the knee in extension are 13 degrees for males and 18 degrees for females. Angles either greater than or less than these norms may be indicative of, but alone are not always accurate in predicting, patellofemoral pathology.

SPECIAL CONSIDERATIONS/COMMENTS

Dynamic Q-angle measurements, where the subject is standing and the quadriceps muscle is in a contracted state, may be more indicative of patellofemoral function and underlying lower extremity pathomechanics than static Q-angle measurements. The accuracy of the Q-angle measurement has come into question. The proximal attachment of the rectus femoris muscle is the anterior inferior iliac spines and not the anterior superior iliac spines. This may provide for an invalid measurement because the anterior inferior iliac spines do not appear to fall in line between the anterior superior iliac spines and the mid-patella.

EVIDENCE

	Greene et al (2001)
Study design	Reliability
Conditions evaluated	Patellar malalignment
Sample size	25
Reliability	Interobserver reliability: .17 to .29 Intraobserver reliability: .14 to .37
Sensitivity	Not evaluated
Specificity	Not evaluated

REFERENCES

Bayraktar B, Yucesir I, Ozturk A, et al. Change of quadriceps angle values with age and activity. *Saudi Med J.* 2004;25(6):756-760.

Biedert RM, Warnke K. Correlation between the Q angle and the patella position: a clinical and axial computed tomography evaluation. *Arch Orthop Trauma Surg.* 2001;121(6):346-349.

France L, Nester C. Effect of errors in the identification of anatomical landmarks on the accuracy of Q angle values. *Clin Biomech (Bristol, Avon).* 2001; 16(8):710-713.

Greene CC, Edwards TB, Wade MR, Carson EW. Reliability of the quadriceps angle measurement. *Am J Knee Surg.* 2001;14(2):97-103.

Guerra JP, Arnold MJ, Gajdosik RL. Q angle: effects of isometric quadriceps contraction and body position. *J Orthop Sports Phys Ther.* 1994;19(4):200-204.

Herrington L, Nester C. Q-angle undervalued? The relationship between Q-angle and medio-lateral position of the patella. *Clin Biomech (Bristol, Avon).* 2004;19(10):1070-1073.

Horton MG, Hall TL. Quadriceps femoris muscle angle: normal values and relationships with gender and selected skeletal measures. *Phys Ther.* 1989; 69(11):897-901.

Hvid I, Andersen LI. The quadriceps angle and its relation to femoral torsion. *Acta Orthop Scand.* 1982;53(4):577-579.

Lathinghouse LH, Trimble MH. Effects of isometric quadriceps activation on the Q-angle in women before and after quadriceps exercise. *J Orthop Sports Phys Ther.* 2000;30(4):211-216.

Livingston LA. The accuracy of Q angle values. *Clin Biomech (Bristol, Avon).* 2002;17(4):322-323; author reply 323-324.

Olerud C, Berg P. The variation of the Q angle with different positions of the foot. *Clin Orthop Relat Res.* 1984;(191):162-165.

Tomsich DA, Nitz AJ, Threlkeld AJ, Shapiro R. Patellofemoral alignment: reliability. *J Orthop Sports Phys Ther.* 1996;23(3):200-208.

Woodland LH, Francis RS. Parameters and comparisons of the quadriceps angle of college-aged men and women in the supine and standing positions. *Am J Sports Med.* 1992;20(2):208-211.

KNEE

MEDIAL-LATERAL GRIND TEST

TEST POSITIONING

The subject lies supine. The examiner stands next to the involved side and holds the subject's foot. The examiner's other hand is placed over the joint line of the knee (Figure K10-6A).

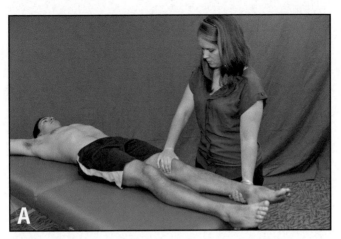

Figure K10-6A.

ACTION

The examiner passively flexes the subject's hip and knee maximally (Figure K10-6B) and then applies a circular motion with the tibia, rotating the tibia clockwise and counterclockwise (Figure K10-6C).

POSITIVE FINDING

Pain, grinding, or clicking is indicative of a meniscal tear.

KNEE

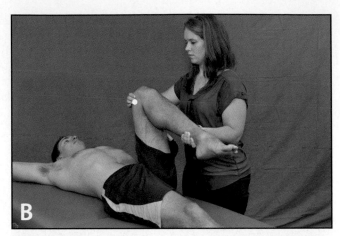

Figure K10-6B.

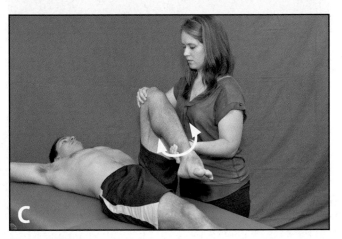

Figure K10-6C.

SPECIAL CONSIDERATIONS/COMMENTS

Varus and valgus stress may be simultaneously applied by the hand over the joint line as the knee is passively extended (Anderson Medial-Lateral Grind Test).

REFERENCE

Anderson AF, Lipscomb AB. Clinical diagnosis of meniscal tears: description of a new manipulative test. *Am J Sports Med*. 1986;14(4):291-293.

BOUNCE HOME TEST

TEST POSITIONING

The subject lies supine. The examiner stands next to the involved side and cups the subject's foot in one hand. The examiner's other hand may be placed over the joint line of the knee (Figure K10-7A).

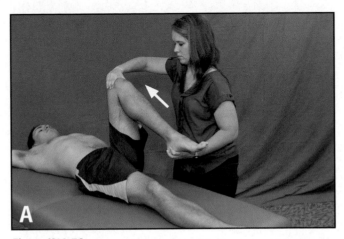

Figure K10-7A.

ACTION

The examiner passively flexes the subject's knee and then allows the knee to passively fall into extension (Figure K10-7B).

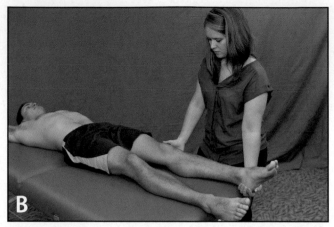

Figure K10-7B.

POSITIVE FINDING

A rubbery endfeel or springy block is indicative of a meniscal tear.

SPECIAL CONSIDERATIONS/COMMENTS

This test should be performed with caution when suspicion of a meniscal tear exists because it may not be comfortable to the patient and could potentially cause further internal derangement.

REFERENCE

Smith BW, Green GA. Acute knee injuries: part I. History and physical examination. *Am Fam Physician.* 1995;51(3):615-621.

KNEE

PATELLAR GRIND TEST (CLARKE'S SIGN)

TEST POSITIONING

The subject lies supine with the knees extended. The examiner stands next to the involved side and places the web space of the thumb on the superior border of the patella (Figure K10-8A).

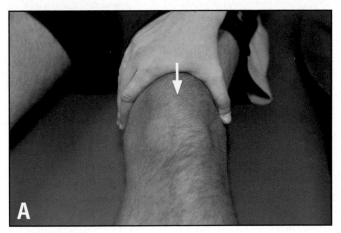

Figure K10-8A.

ACTION

The subject is asked to contract the quadriceps muscle while the examiner applies downward and inferior pressure on the patella (Figure K10-8B).

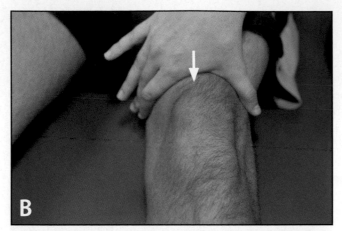

Figure K10-8B. Note: The patient actively contracts the quadriceps muscle while the examiner applies a gentle downward pressure on the patella.

POSITIVE FINDING

Pain with movement of the patella or an inability to complete the test is indicative of chondromalacia patella.

SPECIAL CONSIDERATIONS/COMMENTS

This test may be painful even for healthy subjects; therefore, it is important to bilaterally compare. This test may be repeated with the subject's knee in 30 and 60 degrees of flexion to assess varying surfaces of the patella. From an objective perspective, chondromalacia can be detected only with surgical intervention because it refers to a softening of the cartilage on the undersurface of the patella that is found with direct palpation.

EVIDENCE

	Cook et al (2012)
Study design	Systematic review
Conditions evaluated	Patellar femoral pain syndrome
Study number	4
Reliability	Not evaluated
Sensitivity	29 to 49
Specificity	67 to 95

REFERENCES

Cook C, Mabry L, Reiman MP, Hegedus EJ. Best tests/clinical findings for screening and diagnosis of patellofemoral pain syndrome: a systematic review. *Physiotherapy.* 2012;98(2):93-100.

Fowler PJ, Lubliner JA. The predictive value of five clinical signs in the evaluation of meniscal pathology. *Arthroscopy.* 1989;5(3):184-186.

Smith BW, Green GA. Acute knee injuries: part I. History and physical examination. *Am Fam Physician.* 1995;51(3):615-621.

KNEE

RENNE TEST

TEST POSITIONING

The subject stands. The examiner stands in front of the subject and places 2 fingers or the thumb over the lateral epicondyle of the involved knee (Figure K10-9A).

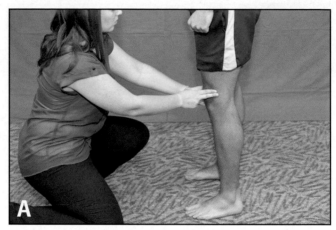

Figure K10-9A. Note that the examiner is applying pressure over the lateral epicondyle of the femur while the subject stands with the knee in full extension.

ACTION

The subject is instructed to support the body weight on the involved foot and actively flex the knee as if performing a squat. The examiner maintains pressure with the thumb over the lateral epicondyle (Figure K10-9B).

KNEE

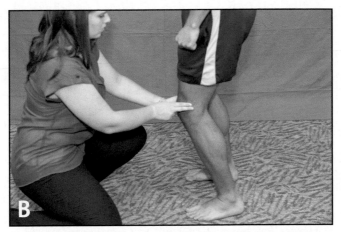

Figure K10-9B. Note that the examiner is applying pressure over the lateral epicondyle of the femur while the subject flexes the knee.

POSITIVE FINDING

If pain is present under the examiner's thumb when the subject's knee is positioned in 30 degrees of flexion, iliotibial band friction syndrome is indicated.

SPECIAL CONSIDERATIONS/COMMENTS

At 30 degrees of knee flexion, the iliotibial band lies directly over the lateral epicondyle. This is an active, weight-bearing version of the Noble test.

REFERENCES

Kirk KL, Kuklo T, Klemme W. Iliotibial band friction syndrome. *Orthopedics.* 2000;23(11):1209-1214.

Renne JW. The iliotibial band friction syndrome. *J Bone Joint Surg.* 1975;57A(8):1110-1111.

KNEE

Noble Test

Test Positioning

The subject lies supine with the knee flexed up to 90 degrees. The examiner stands on the involved side and places the thumb over the lateral epicondyle of the involved knee. The other hand is placed around the subject's ankle.

Action

The examiner passively flexes and extends the subject's knee while maintaining pressure over the lateral epicondyle (Figures K10-10A and K10-10B). Note that the figures are taken from the uninvolved side to better show hand placement.

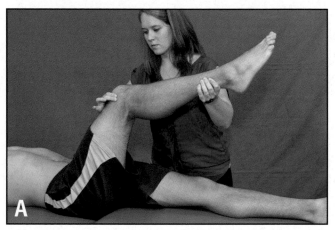

Figure K10-10A. Note that the examiner's fingers are over the lateral epicondyle of the femur.

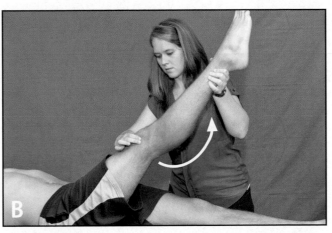

Figure K10-10B.

Positive Finding

If pain is present under the examiner's thumb when the subject's knee is positioned in 30 degrees of flexion, iliotibial band friction syndrome is indicated.

Special Considerations/Comments

At 30 degrees of knee flexion, the iliotibial band lies directly over the lateral epicondyle. This is a passive, nonweightbearing version of the Renne test.

Reference

Calmbach WL, Hutchens M. Evaluation of patients presenting with knee pain: part II. Differential diagnosis. *Am Fam Physician.* 2003;68:917-922.

KNEE

HUGHSTON'S PLICA TEST

TEST POSITIONING

The subject lies supine with the involved knee extended and relaxed. The examiner stands on the involved side and places the heel of one hand over the lateral border of the patella, with the fingers of that hand positioned over the medial femoral condyle. The examiner's other hand is placed around the subject's ankle and foot (Figure K10-11A).

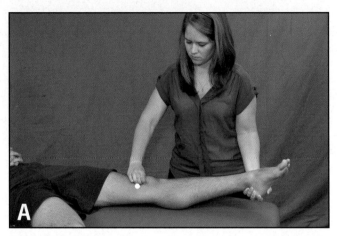

Figure K10-11A.

ACTION

The examiner passively flexes and extends the subject's knee while simultaneously internally rotating the tibia and pushing the patella medially (Figure K10-11B).

POSITIVE FINDING

Pain and/or popping over the medial aspect of the knee is indicative of an abnormal plica. Plica bands may be present and asymptomatic in an otherwise healthy individual. Thus, the location of the band will determine whether patella tracking will be affected.

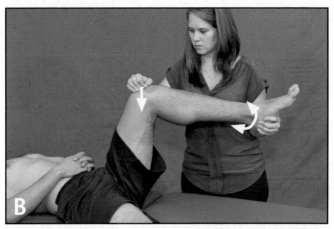

Figure K10-11B.

SPECIAL CONSIDERATIONS/COMMENTS

An aggressive approach to assessing an inflamed plica may lead to further irritation of the structure.

REFERENCES

Eren OT. The accuracy of joint line tenderness by physical examination in the diagnosis of meniscal tears. *Arthroscopy.* 2003;19(8):850-854.

Hughston JC, Whatley GS, Dodelin RA, Stone MM. The role of the supra-patellar plica in internal derangement of the knee. *Am J Orthop.* 1963;5:25-257.

Irha E, Vrdoljak J. Medial synovial plica syndrome of the knee: a diagnostic pitfall in adolescent athletes. *J Pediatr Orthop B.* 2003;12(1):44-48.

Kim SJ, Jeong JH, Cheon YM, Ryu SW. MPP test in the diagnosis of medial patellar plica syndrome. *Arthroscopy.* 2004;20(10):1101-1103.

Zeren B, Oztekin HH. Symptomatic "bucket-handle tear" of the medial patellar plicae in three patients: congenital or acquired? *Am J Sports Med.* 2004;32:1748-1750.

Zhao E, Dai J, Chen D, Lin H. Clinical diagnostic standard of mediopatellar plica syndrome [article in Chinese]. *Zhonghua Wai Ke Za Zhi.* 1998;36(6):355-735.

KNEE

GODFREY 90/90 TEST

TEST POSITIONING

The subject lies supine on a table with both the hip and knee of the involved side flexed to 90 degrees.

ACTION

The examiner passively stabilizes the positioning of the subject's hip and knee while assessing the location of the tibia along the longitudinal axis (Figure K10-12).

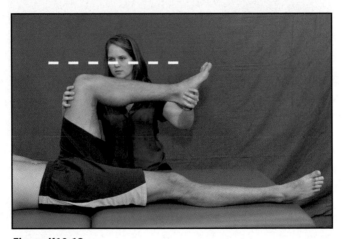

Figure K10-12.

POSITIVE FINDING

The recognition of one tibia resting more inferiorly than the contralateral side may indicate a posterior sag or instability. This may be related to the posterior cruciate ligament (PCL).

SPECIAL CONSIDERATIONS/COMMENTS

This test must be performed bilaterally. Applying a superior force to the tibia from the posterior aspect may reduce the alignment to a normal resting position if it is actually found to be sagging. It is important to maintain neutral tibial rotation, otherwise a positive finding may be the result of a capsular extensibility.

POSTERIOR SAG TEST (GRAVITY DRAWER TEST)

TEST POSITIONING

The subject lies on a table with the involved knee flexed to 90 degrees and the ipsilateral hip placed in 45 degrees of flexion (Figure K10-13). The sole of the subject's foot should be placed on the table.

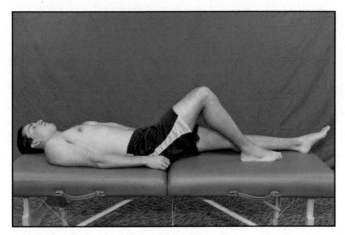

Figure K10-13.

ACTION

The examiner observes the position of the tibia relative to the femur in the sagittal plane. The examiner then instructs the subject to actively contract the quadriceps muscle group in an attempt to extend the knee while retaining hip flexion. The ipsilateral foot should remain on the table during the attempted knee extension.

POSITIVE FINDING

Posterior displacement of the tibia on the femur while the subject's quadriceps remain silent indicates a posterior instability. This may be reflective of injury to any of the following structures: PCL, arcuate ligament complex, and posterior oblique ligament.

KNEE

SPECIAL CONSIDERATIONS/COMMENTS

It is imperative for the examiner to identify a neutral tibiofemoral joint position because this test can be misinterpreted for an anterior instability when one observes an anterior translation of the tibia on the femur.

EVIDENCE

	Malanga et al (2003)
Study design	Systematic review
Conditions evaluated	PCL injuries
Study number	1
Reliability	Not evaluated
Sensitivity	79
Specificity	100

REFERENCES

Akisue T, Kurosaka M, Yoshiya S, Kuroda R, Mizuno K. Evaluation of healing of the injured posterior cruciate ligament: analysis of instability and magnetic resonance imaging. *Arthroscopy*. 2001;17(3):264-269.

Giffin JR, Vogrin TM, Zantop T, Woo SL, Harner CD. Effects of increasing tibial slope on the biomechanics of the knee. *Am J Sports Med*. 2004;32(2):376-382.

Malanga GA, Andrus S, Nadler SF, McLean J. Physical examination of the knee: a review of the original test description and scientific validity of common orthopedic tests. *Arch Phys Med Rehabil*. 2003;84(4):592-603.

Ogata K, McCarthy JA, Dunlap J, Manske PR. Pathomechanics of posterior sag of the tibia in posterior cruciate deficient knees. An experimental study. *Am J Sports Med*. 1988;16(6):630-636.

Shino K, Mitsuoka T, Horibe S, Hamada M, Nakata K, Nakamura N. The gravity sag view: a simple radiographic technique to show posterior laxity of the knee. *Arthroscopy*. 2000;16(6):670-672.

Strobel MJ, Weiler A, Schulz MS, Russe K, Eichhorn HJ. Fixed posterior subluxation in posterior cruciate ligament-deficient knees: diagnosis and treatment of a new clinical sign. *Am J Sports Med*. 2002;30(1):32-38.

KNEE

REVERSE PIVOT SHIFT (JAKOB TEST)

TEST POSITIONING

The subject lies supine with the test knee in 40 to 50 degrees of flexion. The examiner stands with the proximal hand on the subject's posterolateral leg, just distal to the patella, with the thumb on or anterior to the fibular head. The distal hand grasps the subject's mid-foot and heel (Figure K10-14A).

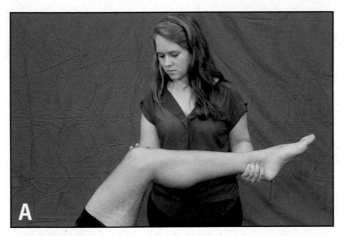

Figure K10-14A.

ALTERNATE TEST POSITIONING

Place the subject's foot between the examiner's distal arm and body, with the same hand on the tibia. The proximal hand should be placed on the posterolateral leg just distal to the knee, with the thumb on or anterior to the fibular head (Figure K10-14B).

KNEE

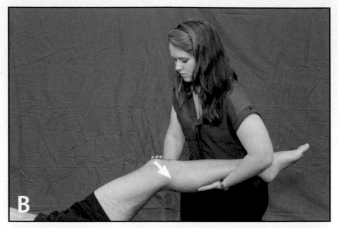

Figure K10-14B.

ACTION

The examiner externally rotates the tibia with one hand and applies a valgus force with the other hand while slowly extending the knee. The same procedure applies for the alternate test position, except a slight axial load is applied as the knee is extended (Figure K10-14C).

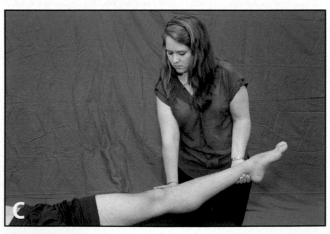

Figure K10-14C.

Positive Finding

This is first seen when the examiner flexes the subject's knee if the lateral tibial plateau subluxes posteriorly. Furthermore, this subluxation is reduced once the knee extends and approaches a position of approximately 20 degrees of flexion. At this point, the lateral tibial plateau will return to a neutral position. A palpable "clunk" or shift as it approaches extension (~20 to 30 degrees of flexion) is indicative of posterolateral rotary instability secondary to damage of primarily the PCL, lateral collateral ligament (LCL), posterolateral capsule, and arcuate complex.

Special Considerations/Comments

This test is very sensitive for the subject who possesses an instability. It should be performed only with the subject relaxed because as a contraction of the surrounding musculature of the knee may prevent a subtle subluxation and indicate a negative test.

Evidence

	Rubinstein et al (1994)
Study design	Randomized controlled trial
Conditions evaluated	PCL injuries
Sample size	39
Reliability	Not evaluated
Sensitivity	26
Specificity	95

KNEE

References

Jakob RP, Hassler H, Staeubli HU. Observations on rotary instability of the lateral compartment of the knee. *Acta Orthop Scand Suppl.* 1981;52(Suppl 191):1-32.

LaPrade RF, Muench C, Wentorf F, Lewis JL. The effect of injury to the posterolateral structures of the knee on force in a posterior cruciate ligament graft: a biomechanical study. *Am J Sports Med.* 2002;30:233-238.

LaPrade RF, Terry GC. Injuries to the posterolateral aspect of the knee: association of anatomic injury patterns with clinical instability. *Am J Sports Med.* 1997;25(4):433-438.

Nielsen S, Helmig P. Posterior instability of the knee joint. An experimental study. *Arch Orthop Trauma Surg.* 1986;105(2):121-125.

Rubinstein RA Jr, Shelbourne KD, McCarroll JR, VanMeter CD, Rettig AC. The accuracy of the clinical examination in the setting of posterior cruciate ligament injuries. *Am J Sports Med.* 1994;22(4):550-557.

ANTERIOR LACHMAN'S TEST

TEST POSITIONING

The subject lies supine with the test knee flexed to 20 to 30 degrees. The examiner stands with the proximal hand on the subject's distal thigh (laterally) immediately proximal to the patella and the distal hand on the subject's proximal tibia (medially) immediately distal to the tibial tubercle (Figure K10-15A).

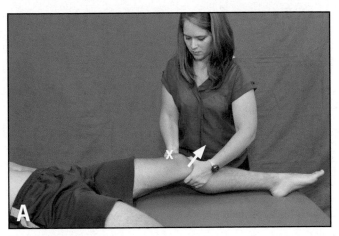

Figure K10-15A.

ALTERNATE TEST POSITIONING

The examiner places his or her flexed knee under the patient's test knee, with the proximal hand over the distal thigh (anteriorly) and distal hand on the subject's proximal tibia (medially), just distal to the tibial tubercle (Figure K10-15B).

KNEE

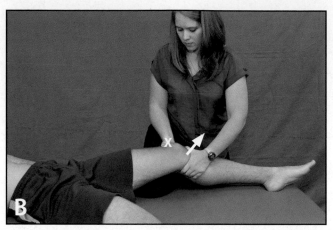

Figure K10-15B.

ACTION

From a "neutral" (anterior-posterior) position, apply an anterior force to the tibia with the distal hand while stabilizing the femur with the proximal hand. The same procedure applies for the alternate test positioning.

POSITIVE FINDING

Excessive anterior translation of the tibia compared to the uninvolved knee with a diminished or absent endpoint is indicative of a partial or complete tear of the anterior cruciate ligament (ACL).

SPECIAL CONSIDERATIONS/COMMENTS

Increased anterior tibial translation is not in and of itself indicative of ACL pathology. For example, a torn PCL will allow the proximal tibia to translate posteriorly, thus producing increased anterior translation during the anterior Lachman's test. Meniscal tear (primarily of the posterior horn) may also contribute to an anterior translation. Therefore, the presence and quality of the endpoint must be determined before ACL integrity can be accurately assessed. Although individuals may choose to always use the dominant hand for the translation assessment, it is recommended to stabilize the tibia on the medial side to prevent the possibility of increased external rotation of the tibia, which can contribute to increased anterior translation.

KNEE

EVIDENCE

	Benjaminse et al (2006)	van Eck et al (2013)
Study design	Meta-analysis	Meta-analysis
Conditions evaluated	ACL injuries	ACL ruptures
Study number	21	18
Reliability	Not evaluated	Not evaluated
Sensitivity	85	81
Specificity	94	81

REFERENCES

Benjaminse A, Gokeler A, van der Schans CP. Clinical diagnosis of an anterior cruciate ligament rupture: a meta-analysis. *J Orthop Sports Phys Ther.* 2006;36(5):267-288.

Cooperman JM, Riddle DL, Rothstein JM. Reliability and validity of judgments of the integrity of the ACL of the knee using the Lachman's test. *Phys Ther.* 1990;70:225-233.

Jonsson T, Althoff B, Peterson L, Renström P. Clinical diagnosis of ruptures of the anterior cruciate ligament: a comparative study of the Lachman test and the anterior drawer sign. *Am J Sports Med.* 1982;10(2):100-102.

Kim SJ, Kim HK. Reliability of the anterior drawer test, the pivot shift test, and the Lachman test. *Clin Orthop Relat Res.* 1995;(317):237-242.

Konig DP, Rütt J, Kumm D, Breidenbach E. Diagnosis of anterior knee instability. Comparison between the Lachman test, the KT-1,000 arthrometer and the ultrasound Lachman test [article in German]. *Unfallchirurg.* 1998;101(3):209-213.

Kumar VP, Satku K. The false positive Lachman test. *Singapore Med J.* 1993;34(6):551-552.

Liu W, Maitland ME, Bell GD. A modeling study of partial ACL injury: simulated KT-2000 arthrometer tests. *J Biomech Eng.* 2002;124(3):294-301.

van der Plas CG, Opstelten W, Devillé WL, Bijl D, Bouter LM, Scholten RJ. Physical diagnosis—the value of some common tests for the demonstration of an anterior cruciate-ligament rupture: meta-analysis. *Ned Tijdschr Geneeskd.* 2005;149(2):83-88.

van Eck CF, van den Bekerom MP, Fu FH, Poolman RW, Kerkhoffs GM. Methods to diagnose acute anterior cruciate ligament rupture: a meta-analysis of physical examinations with and without anaesthesia. *Knee Surg Sports Traumatol Arthrosc.* 2013;21(8):1895-1903.

KNEE

ANTERIOR DRAWER TEST

TEST POSITIONING

The subject lies supine with the test hip flexed to 45 degrees, knee flexed to 90 degrees, and foot in neutral position. The examiner sits on the subject's foot with both hands behind the subject's proximal tibia and thumbs on the tibial plateau (Figure K10-16).

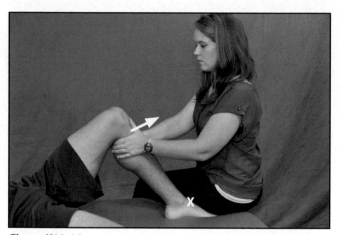

Figure K10-16.

ACTION

Apply an anterior force to the proximal tibia. The hamstring tendons should be palpated frequently with index fingers to ensure relaxation.

POSITIVE FINDING

Increased anterior tibial displacement as compared to the uninvolved side is indicative of a partial or complete tear of the ACL.

SPECIAL CONSIDERATIONS/COMMENTS

See Special Considerations/Comments for the Anterior Lachman's test. Qualitative assessment of the endpoint during the Anterior Drawer Test is less accurate than during the Anterior Lachman's Test.

Also, there is a greater potential for a false-negative finding with this test versus the Anterior Lachman's Test, secondary to the increased potential for hamstring "guarding."

EVIDENCE

	Benjaminse et al (2006)	van Eck et al (2013)
Study design	Meta-analysis	Meta-analysis
Conditions evaluated	ACL injuries	ACL rupture
Study number	20	15
Reliability	Not evaluated	Not evaluated
Sensitivity	55	38
Specificity	92	81

REFERENCES

Benjaminse A, Gokeler A, van der Schans CP. Clinical diagnosis of an anterior cruciate ligament rupture: a meta-analysis. *J Orthop Sports Phys Ther.* 2006;36(5):267-288.

Graham GP, Johnson S, Dent CM, Fairclough JA. Comparison of clinical tests and the KT1000 in the diagnosis of anterior cruciate ligament rupture. *Br J Sports Med.* 1991;25(2):96-97.

Johnson MW. Acute knee effusions: a systematic approach to diagnosis. *Am Fam Physician.* 2000;61(8):2391-2400.

Jonsson T, Althoff B, Peterson L, Renström P. Clinical diagnosis of ruptures of the anterior cruciate ligament: a comparative study of the Lachman test and the anterior drawer sign. *Am J Sports Med.* 1982;10(2):100-102.

Kim SJ, Kim HK. Reliability of the anterior drawer test, the pivot shift test, and the Lachman test. *Clin Orthop Relat Res.* 1995;(317):237-242.

van der Plas CG, Opstelten W, Devillé WL, Bijl D, Bouter LM, Scholten RJ. Physical diagnosis—the value of some common tests for the demonstration of an anterior cruciate-ligament rupture: meta-analysis. *Ned Tijdschr Geneeskd.* 2005;149(2):83-88.

van Eck CF, van den Bekerom MP, Fu FH, Poolman RW, Kerkhoffs GM. Methods to diagnose acute anterior cruciate ligament rupture: a meta-analysis of physical examinations with and without anaesthesia. *Knee Surg Sports Traumatol Arthrosc.* 2013;21(8):1895-1903.

SLOCUM TEST WITH INTERNAL TIBIAL ROTATION

TEST POSITIONING

The subject lies supine with the test hip flexed to 45 degrees, knee flexed to 90 degrees, and tibia internally rotated 15 to 20 degrees. The examiner sits on the subject's foot with both hands behind the subject's proximal tibia and thumbs on the tibial plateau (Figure K10-17).

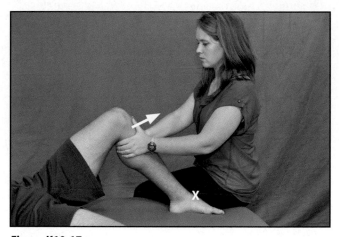

Figure K10-17.

ACTION

Apply an anterior force to the proximal tibia. The hamstring tendons should be palpated frequently with the index fingers to ensure relaxation.

POSITIVE FINDING

Increased anterior tibial displacement, particularly of the lateral tibial condyle, as compared to the uninvolved side is indicative of anterolateral rotary instability (secondary to a partial or complete tear of primarily the ACL and posterolateral capsule).

KNEE

Special Considerations/Comments

The examiner must avoid maximally rotating the tibia because this will tighten most of the surrounding structures and create a high potential for false-negative findings.

References

Anderson AF, Rennirt GW, Standeffer WC Jr. Clinical analysis of the pivot shift tests: description of the pivot drawer test. *Am J Knee Surg.* 2000;13(1):19-23; discussion 23-24.

Slocum DB, James SI, Larson RI, Singer KM. A clinical test for anterolateral rotary instability of the knee. *Clin Orthop.* 1976;118:63-69.

Slocum DB, Larson RI. Rotatory instability of the knee. *J Bone Joint Surg Am.* 1968;50(2):211-215.

SLOCUM TEST WITH EXTERNAL TIBIAL ROTATION

TEST POSITIONING

The subject lies supine with the test hip flexed to 45 degrees, knee flexed to 90 degrees, and tibia externally rotated 15 to 20 degrees. The examiner sits on the subject's foot with both hands behind the subject's proximal tibia and thumbs on the tibial plateau (Figure K10-18).

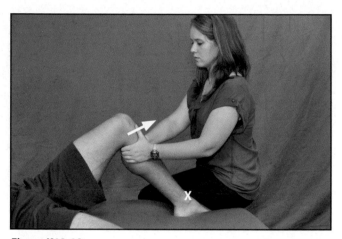

Figure K10-18.

ACTION

Apply an anterior force to the proximal tibia. The hamstring tendons should be palpated frequently with the index fingers to ensure relaxation.

POSITIVE FINDING

Increased anterior tibial displacement, particularly of the medial tibial condyle, compared to the uninvolved side is indicative of anteromedial rotary instability secondary to damage to primarily the medial collateral ligament (MCL), ACL, and posteromedial capsule.

KNEE

SPECIAL CONSIDERATIONS/COMMENTS

The examiner must avoid maximally rotating the tibia because this will tighten most of the surrounding structures and create a high potential for false-negative findings.

REFERENCES

Anderson AF, Rennirt GW, Standeffer WC Jr. Clinical analysis of the pivot shift tests: description of the pivot drawer test. *Am J Knee Surg.* 2000;13(1):19-23.

Slocum DB, Larson RI. Rotatory instability of the knee. *J Bone Joint Surg Am.* 1968;50(2):211-215.

Pivot Shift Test

Test Positioning

The subject lies supine with the test knee in full extension. The examiner stands with the proximal hand on the subject's anterolateral tibiofemoral joint, with the thumb on or posterior to the fibular head. The distal hand grasps the subject's midfoot and heel (Figure K10-19A).

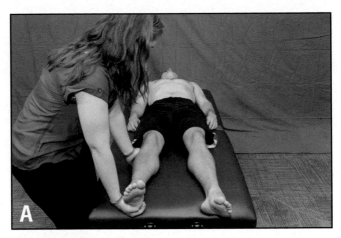

Figure K10-19A.

Alternate Test Positioning

Place the subject's foot between the examiner's distal arm and body with the same hand on the tibia. The proximal hand is placed on the posterolateral leg, just distal to the knee, with the thumb on or posterior to the fibular head (Figure K10-19B).

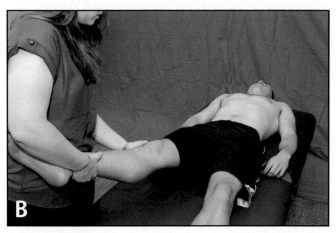

Figure K10-19B.

ACTION

Internally rotate the tibia with the distal hand, apply a valgus force with the proximal hand, and slowly flex the knee (Figure K10-19C). The same procedure applies for the alternate test positioning, except a slight axial load is first applied to the extended knee.

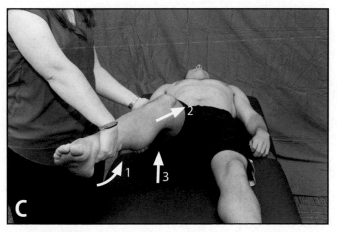

Figure K10-19C.

POSITIVE FINDING

A palpable "clunk" or shift at ~20 to 30 degrees of flexion is indicative of anterolateral rotary instability secondary to tearing of the ACL and posterolateral capsule.

SPECIAL CONSIDERATIONS/COMMENTS

It is important to provide the axial load before flexing the knee, as this helps to accentuate the "clunk" or shift that will facilitate detection of a trace pivot shift. It should be noted that this test often reproduces the mechanism of injury, which may create subject anxiety and apprehension, thus increasing the potential for false-negative findings. This may be the most sensitive and accurate test for assessing anterior tibiofemoral instability. However, it is difficult to perform and subject anxiety reduces the opportunity for the clinician to gain experience as compared to administering other special tests.

EVIDENCE

	Benjaminse et al (2006)	van Eck et al (2013)
Study design	Meta-analysis	Meta-analysis
Conditions evaluated	ACL injuries	ACL ruptures
Study number	15	14
Reliability	Not evaluated	Not evaluated
Sensitivity	24	28
Specificity	98	81

REFERENCES

Anderson AF, Rennirt GW, Standeffer WC Jr. Clinical analysis of the pivot shift tests: description of the pivot drawer test. *Am J Knee Surg.* 2000;13(1):19-23.

Benjaminse A, Gokeler A, van der Schans CP. Clinical diagnosis of an anterior cruciate ligament rupture: a meta-analysis. *J Orthop Sports Phys Ther.* 2006;36(5):267-288.

Kim SJ, Kim HK. Reliability of the anterior drawer test, the pivot shift test, and the Lachman test. *Clin Orthop Relat Res.* 1995;(317):237-242.

van der Plas CG, Opstelten W, Deville WL, Bijl D, Bouter LM, Scholten RJ. Physical diagnosis—the value of some common tests for the demonstration of an anterior cruciate-ligament rupture: meta-analysis. *Ned Tijdschr Geneeskd.* 2005;149(2):83-88.

van Eck CF, van den Bekerom MP, Fu FH, Poolman RW, Kerkhoffs GM. Methods to diagnose acute anterior cruciate ligament rupture: a meta-analysis of physical examinations with and without anaesthesia. *Knee Surg Sports Traumatol Arthrosc.* 2013;21(8):1895-1903.

KNEE

JERK TEST

TEST POSITIONING

The subject lies supine with the involved hip flexed to 45 degrees. The examiner stands next to the involved side and holds the subject's foot. The examiner's other hand is placed over the lateral aspect of the knee, just behind the head of the fibula (Figure K10-20A). The knee may be slightly flexed. (Note: Another perk of the accompanying video is that some of the 2-dimensional photos are hard to decipher between in still images.)

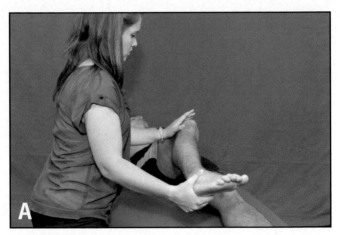

Figure K10-20A.

ACTION

The examiner passively flexes the subject's knee to 90 degrees (Figure K10-20B). Then the examiner extends the subject's knee while applying a valgus force and internally rotating the tibia (Figure K10-20C).

KNEE

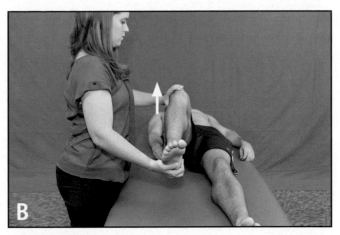

Figure K10-20B.

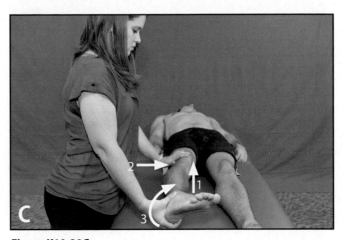

Figure K10-20C.

POSITIVE FINDING

A shift or "clunk" felt at 30 degrees of knee flexion while the knee is being extended indicates a positive test, implicating anterolateral rotary instability. If a shift is present, it will reduce on further passive extension of the knee.

SPECIAL CONSIDERATIONS/COMMENTS

This test may not be as sensitive as the Pivot Shift Test.

REFERENCES

Dupont JY, Bellier G. The jerk-test in external rotation in rupture of the anterior cruciate ligament. Description and significance [article in French]. *Rev Chir Orthop Reparatrice Appar Mot.* 1988;74(5):413-423.

Graham GP, Johnson S, Dent CM, Fairclough JA. Comparison of clinical tests and the KT1000 in the diagnosis of anterior cruciate ligament rupture. *Br J Sports Med.* 1991;25(2):96-97.

POSTERIOR DRAWER TEST

TEST POSITIONING

The subject lies supine with the test hip flexed to 45 degrees, knee flexed to 90 degrees, and foot in neutral position. The examiner sits on the subject's foot with both hands behind the subject's proximal tibia and thumbs on the tibial plateau (Figure K10-21).

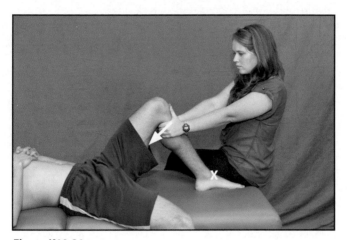

Figure K10-21.

ACTION

Apply a posterior force to the proximal tibia.

POSITIVE FINDING

Increased posterior tibial displacement as compared to the uninvolved side is indicative of a partial or complete tear of the PCL.

SPECIAL CONSIDERATIONS/COMMENTS

It is important to maintain quadriceps and hamstring muscle relaxation during this test. While applying a posterior force, the examiner should carefully assess any posterior "step-off" from the tibial plateau on the femur.

KNEE

EVIDENCE

	Malanga et al (2003)
Study design	Systematic review
Conditions evaluated	PCL injuries
Study number	6
Reliability	Not evaluated
Sensitivity	51 to 90
Specificity	99

REFERENCES

Hughston JC. The absent posterior drawer test in some acute posterior cruciate ligament tears of the knee. *Am J Sports Med*. 1988;16(1):39-43.

Logan M, Williams A, Lavelle J, Gedroyc W, Freeman M. The effect of posterior cruciate ligament deficiency on knee kinematics. *Am J Sports Med*. 2004;32(8):1915-1922.

Malanga GA, Andrus S, Nadler SF, McLean J. Physical examination of the knee: a review of the original test description and scientific validity of common orthopedic tests. *Arch Phys Med Rehabil*. 2003;84(4):592-603.

Ritchie JR, Bergfeld JA, Kambic H, Manning T. Isolated sectioning of the medial and posteromedial capsular ligaments in the posterior cruciate ligament-deficient knee: influence on posterior tibial translation. *Am J Sports Med*. 1998;26(3):389-394.

KNEE

HUGHSTON POSTEROMEDIAL DRAWER TEST

TEST POSITIONING

The subject lies supine with the test hip flexed to 45 degrees, knee flexed to 90 degrees, and tibia internally rotated 20 to 30 degrees. The examiner sits on the subject's foot with both hands behind the subject's proximal tibia and thumbs on the tibial plateau (Figure K10-22).

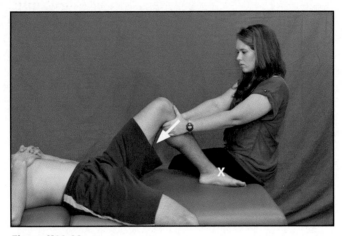

Figure K10-22.

ACTION

Apply a posterior force to the proximal tibia.

POSITIVE FINDING

Increased posterior tibial displacement, particularly of the medial tibial condyle, compared to the uninvolved side is indicative of posteromedial rotary instability (secondary to damage of primarily the PCL, posteromedial capsule, MCL, and posterior oblique ligament).

KNEE

SPECIAL CONSIDERATIONS/COMMENTS

It is important to maintain quadriceps and hamstring muscle relaxation during this test. While applying a posterior force, the examiner should carefully assess any posterior "step-off" from the tibial plateau on the femur.

REFERENCES

Anderson AF, Rennirt GW, Standeffer WC Jr. Clinical analysis of the pivot shift tests: description of the pivot drawer test. *Am J Knee Surg.* 2000;13(1):19-23.

Hughston JC. The absent posterior drawer test in some acute posterior cruciate ligament tears of the knee. *Am J Sports Med.* 1988;16(1):39-43.

Hughston JC, Andrews JR, Cross MJ, Moschi A. The classification of knee ligament instabilities. I. The medical compartment and cruciate ligaments. *J Bone Joint Surg Am.* 1976;58(2):159-172.

HUGHSTON POSTEROLATERAL DRAWER TEST

TEST POSITIONING

The subject lies supine with the test hip flexed to 45 degrees, knee flexed to 90 degrees, and tibia externally rotated 20 to 30 degrees. The examiner sits on the subject's foot with both hands behind the subject's proximal tibia and thumbs on the tibial plateau (Figure K10-23).

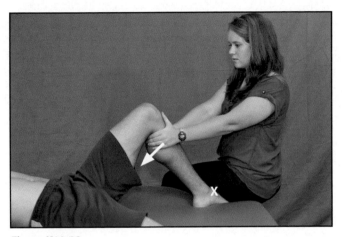

Figure K10-23.

ACTION

Apply a posterior force to the proximal tibia.

POSITIVE FINDING

Increased posterior tibial displacement, particularly of the lateral tibial condyle, compared to the uninvolved side is indicative of posterolateral rotary instability (secondary to damage of the PCL, LCL, posterolateral capsule, and arcuate complex).

KNEE

SPECIAL CONSIDERATIONS/COMMENTS

It is important to maintain quadriceps and hamstring muscle relaxation during this test. While applying a posterior force, the examiner should carefully assess any posterior "step-off" from the tibial plateau on the femur.

REFERENCES

Anderson AF, Rennirt GW, Standeffer WC Jr. Clinical analysis of the pivot shift tests: description of the pivot drawer test. *Am J Knee Surg.* 2000;13(1):19-23.

Hughston JC. The absent posterior drawer test in some acute posterior cruciate ligament tears of the knee. *Am J Sports Med.* 1988;16(1):39-43.

Hughston JC, Andrews JR, Cross MJ, Moschi A. The classification of knee ligament instabilities. I. The medical compartment and cruciate ligaments. *J Bone Joint Surg Am.* 1976;58(2):159-172.

Hughston JC, Norwood LA Jr. The posterolateral drawer and external rotation recurvatum test for posterolateral rotatory instability of the knee. *Clin Orthop Relat Res.* 1980;(147):82-87.

POSTERIOR LACHMAN'S TEST

TEST POSITIONING

The subject lies supine with the test knee flexed to 20 to 30 degrees. The examiner stands with the proximal hand on the subject's distal thigh (laterally) immediately proximal to the patella and the distal hand on the subject's proximal tibia (medially) immediately distal to the tibial tubercle (Figure K10-24).

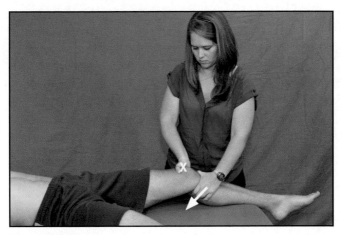

Figure K10-24.

ACTION

From a "neutral" (anterior-posterior) position, apply a posterior force to the tibia with the distal hand while the femur is stabilized with the proximal hand.

POSITIVE FINDING

Excessive posterior translation of the tibia (compared to the uninvolved knee) from the neutral position with a diminished or absent endpoint is indicative of a partial or complete tear of the PCL.

KNEE

Special Considerations/Comments

If the posterior Lachman's test is not performed from a neutral position, the involved knee may actually present with decreased posterior tibial translation compared to the uninvolved knee. This decrease is most likely due to PCL pathology that allows the proximal tibia to translate posteriorly, thus producing decreased posterior translation and subsequent false-negative findings. Therefore, the presence and quality of the endpoint must be determined before PCL integrity may be accurately assessed.

Evidence

	Rubinstein et al (1994)
Study design	Randomized controlled trial
Conditions evaluated	PCL injuries
Sample size	39
Reliability	Not evaluated
Sensitivity	62
Specificity	89

References

Cooperman JM, Riddle DL, Rothstein JM. Reliability and validity of judgments of the integrity of the ACL of the knee using the Lachman's test. *Phys Ther.* 1990;70(4):225-233.

Feltham GT, Albright JP. The diagnosis of PCL injury: literature review and introduction of two novel tests. *Iowa Orthop J.* 2001;21:36-42.

Rubinstein RA Jr, Shelbourne KD, McCarroll JR, VanMeter CD, Rettig AC. The accuracy of the clinical examination in the setting of posterior cruciate ligament injuries. *Am J Sports Med.* 1994;22(4):550-557.

KNEE

EXTERNAL ROTATION RECURVATUM TEST

TEST POSITIONING

The subject lies supine. The examiner stands and grasps a great toe with each hand.

ACTION

Lift both legs off the table (vertically) by the great toes (Figure K10-25).

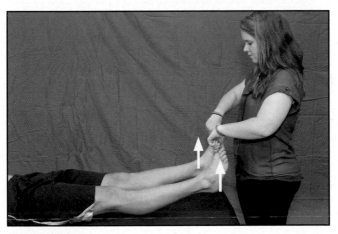

Figure K10-25.

POSITIVE FINDING

An increase in hyperextension and external tibial rotation as compared to the uninvolved knee is indicative of posterolateral rotary instability (secondary to damage of primarily the PCL, LCL, posterolateral capsule, and arcuate complex).

SPECIAL CONSIDERATIONS/COMMENTS

It is important for the examiner to recognize that a positive finding may not be indicative of any pathology and instead may simply be representative of one's normal joint extensibility.

KNEE

EVIDENCE

	Rubinstein et al (1994)
Study design	Randomized controlled trial
Conditions evaluated	PCL injuries
Sample size	39
Reliability	Not evaluated
Sensitivity	3
Specificity	99

REFERENCES

Cooper DE. Tests for posterolateral instability of the knee in normal subjects. Results of examination under anesthesia. *J Bone Joint Surg Am.* 1991;73(1):30-36.

Hughston JC, Norwood LA Jr. The posterolateral drawer test and external rotational recurvatum test for posterolateral rotatory instability of the knee. *Clin Orthop Relat Res.* 1980;147:82-87.

LaPrade RF, Ly TV, Griffith C. The external rotation recurvatum test revisited: reevaluation of the sagittal plane tibiofemoral relationship. *Am J Sports Med.* 2008;36(4):709-712.

LaPrade RF, Wentorf F. Diagnosis and treatment of posterolateral knee injuries. *Clin Orthop Relat Res.* 2002;402:110-121.

Loudon JK, Goist HL, Loudon KL. Genu recurvatum syndrome. *J Orthop Sports Phys Ther.* 1998;27(5):361-367.

Rubinstein RA Jr, Shelbourne KD, McCarroll JR, VanMeter CD, Rettig AC. The accuracy of the clinical examination in the setting of posterior cruciate ligament injuries. *Am J Sports Med.* 1994;22(4):550-557.

Staubli HU, Jakob RP. Posterior instability of the knee near extension. A clinical and stress radiographic analysis of acute injuries of the posterior cruciate ligament. *J Bone Joint Surg Br.* 1990;72(2):225-230.

Trimble MH, Bishop MD, Buckley BD, Fields LC, Rozea GD. The relationship between clinical measurements of lower extremity posture and tibial translation. *Clin Biomech (Bristol, Avon).* 2002;17(4):286-290.

KNEE

DIAL TEST (TIBIAL EXTERNAL ROTATION TEST)

TEST POSITIONING

The subject lies supine with the test knee in 30 degrees flexion and the ankle in neutral plantar flexion/dorsiflexion and inversion/eversion. The examiner grasps the subject's distal thigh (posteriorly) with the proximal hand and the subject's ankle from the plantar surface with the distal hand (Figure K10-26A).

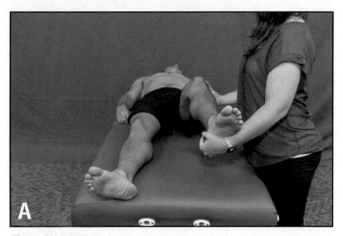

Figure K10-26A.

ACTION

With the proximal hand stabilizing the subject's distal thigh, the examiner maximally externally rotates the subject's lower leg (maintaining the ankle in a neutral position) and measures the amount of external rotation created between the knee and medial border of the foot (Figure K10-26B).

The test is repeated with the knee in 90 degrees of flexion (Figures K10-26C and K10-26D).

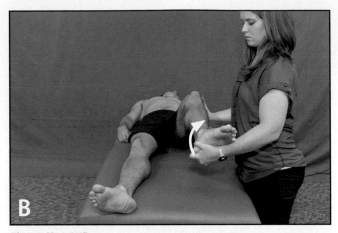

Figure K10-26B.

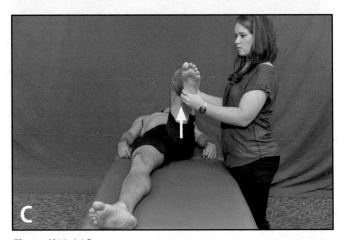

Figure K10-26C.

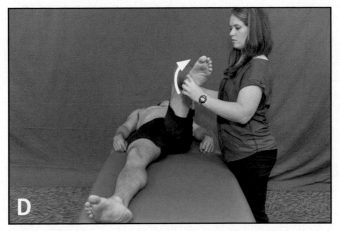

Figure K10-26D.

POSITIVE FINDING

An increase of greater than 10 degrees of external rotation (as compared to the contralateral leg) at 30 degrees but not at 90 degrees is indicative of an isolated posterolateral corner injury. A greater-than-10–degree increase at both angles is indicative of injury to both the posterolateral corner and PCL.

SPECIAL CONSIDERATIONS/COMMENTS

This test can also be performed in the supine position with the knee flexed over the side of the table. It has been proposed that the tibial tubercle be used as the reference point for measuring external rotation because it is a fixed landmark compared to the mobile foot.

KNEE

EVIDENCE

	Krause et al (2013)
Study design	Reliability
Conditions evaluated	External rotation
Sample size	24
Reliability	Intratester (ICC) 30 degrees = .83 to .86 Intratester (ICC) 90 degrees = .87 to .89 Intertester (ICC) 30 degrees = .74 Intertester (ICC) 90 degrees = .83
Sensitivity	Not evaluated
Specificity	Not evaluated

REFERENCES

Bleday RM, Fanelli GC, Giannotti BF, Edson LJ, Barrett TA. Instrumented measurement of the posterolateral corner. *Arthroscopy.* 1998;14(5):489-494.

Cooper DE. Tests for posterolateral instability of the knee in normal subjects. *J Bone Joint Surg Am.* 1991;73(1):30-36.

Dowd GS. Reconstruction of the posterior cruciate ligament. Indications and results. *J Bone Joint Surg Br.* 2004;86(4):480-491.

Krause DA, Levy BA, Shah JP, Stuart MJ, Hollman JH, Dahm DL. Reliability of the dial test using a handheld inclinometer. *Knee Surg Sports Traumatol Arthrosc.* 2013;21(5):1011-1016.

LaPrade RF, Wentorf F. Diagnosis and treatment of posterolateral knee injuries. *Clin Orthop Relat Res.* 2002;(402):110-121.

KNEE

VALGUS STRESS TEST

TEST POSITIONING

The subject lies supine with the knee in full extension (Figure K10-27A). The examiner stands with the distal hand on the subject's medial ankle and the proximal hand on the knee (laterally).

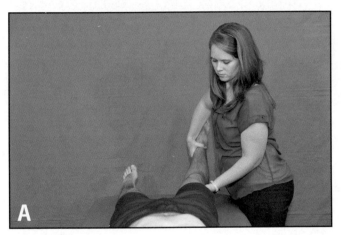

Figure K10-27A.

ACTION

With the ankle stabilized, apply a valgus force at the knee with the proximal hand. This is performed with the knee in full extension and repeated with the knee in 20 to 30 degrees of flexion (Figure K10-27B).

KNEE

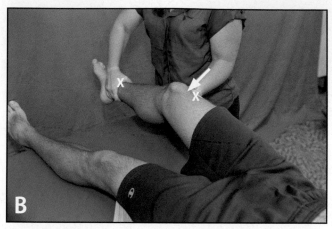

Figure K10-27B.

POSITIVE FINDING

Medial knee pain and/or increased valgus movement with a diminished or absent endpoint as compared to the uninvolved knee is indicative of damage to primarily the MCL, PCL, and posteromedial capsule when found in full extension, and MCL when tested in 20 to 30 degrees of flexion.

SPECIAL CONSIDERATIONS/COMMENTS

The examiner must avoid allowing the femur to internally or externally rotate during this test because this may give the illusion of increased valgus movement. This may be accomplished by using the treatment table to help stabilize the subject's femur (Figure K10-27C).

KNEE

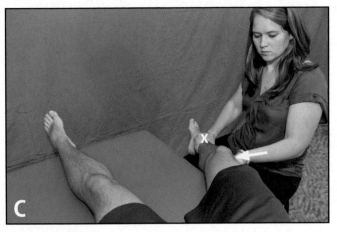

Figure K10-27C.

EVIDENCE

	Malanga et al (2003)
Study design	Systematic review
Conditions evaluated	MCL injuries
Study number	3
Reliability ICC Flexion 30 degrees Full extension	.56 .68
Sensitivity	86 to 96
Specificity	Not evaluated

REFERENCES

Bonifasi-Lista C, Lake SP, Small MS, Weiss JA. Viscoelastic properties of the human medial collateral ligament under longitudinal, transverse and shear loading. *J Orthop Res.* 2005;23(1):67-76.

Malanga GA, Andrus S, Nadler SF, McLean J. Physical examination of the knee: a review of the original test description and scientific validity of common orthopedic tests. *Arch Phys Med Rehabil.* 2003;84(4):592-603.

McClure PW, Rothstein JM, Riddle DL. Intertester reliability of clinical judgments of medial knee ligament integrity. *Phys Ther.* 1989;69(4):268-275.

Nakamura N, Horibe S, Toritsuka Y, Mitsuoka T, Yoshikawa H, Shino K. Acute grade III medial collateral ligament injury of the knee associated with anterior cruciate ligament tear: the usefulness of magnetic resonance imaging in determining a treatment regimen. *Am J Sports Med.* 2003;31(2):261-267.

Sawant M, Narasimha Murty A, Ireland J. Valgus knee injuries: evaluation and documentation using a simple technique of stress radiography. *Knee.* 2004;11(1):25-28.

VARUS STRESS TEST

TEST POSITIONING

The subject lies supine with the knee in full extension (Figure K10-28A). The examiner stands with the distal hand on the subject's lateral ankle and the proximal hand on the knee (medially).

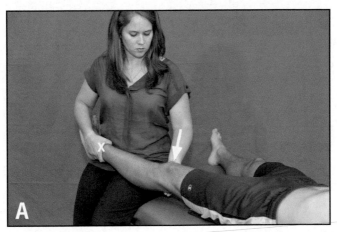

Figure K10-28A.

ACTION

With the ankle stabilized, apply a varus force at the knee with the proximal hand. This is performed with the knee in full extension and repeated with the knee in 20 to 30 degrees of knee flexion (Figure K10-28B).

KNEE

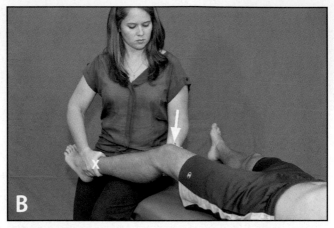

Figure K10-28B.

POSITIVE FINDING

Lateral knee pain and/or increased varus movement with a diminished or absent endpoint as compared to the uninvolved knee is indicative of damage to primarily the LCL, PCL, and arcuate complex when found at full extension, and LCL when tested at 20 to 30 degrees of flexion.

SPECIAL CONSIDERATIONS/COMMENTS

The examiner must avoid allowing the femur to internally or externally rotate during this test because this may give the illusion of increased varus movement. This may be accomplished by using the treatment table to help stabilize the subject's femur (Figure K10-28C).

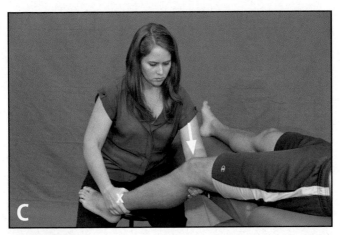

Figure K10-28C.

EVIDENCE

	Malanga et al (2003)
Study design	Meta-analysis
Conditions evaluated	LCL injuries
Study number	1
Reliability	Not evaluated
Sensitivity	25
Specificity	Not evaluated

REFERENCES

Bozkurt M, Yilmaz E, Akseki D, Havitcioğlu H, Günal I. The evaluation of the proximal tibiofibular joint for patients with lateral knee pain. *Knee.* 2004;11(4):307-312.

Hinterwimmer S, Baumgart R, Plitz W. Tension changes in the collateral ligaments of a cruciate ligament-deficient knee joint: an experimental biomechanical study. *Arch Orthop Trauma Surg.* 2002;122(8):454-458.

Malanga GA, Andrus S, Nadler SF, McLean J. Physical examination of the knee: a review of the original test description and scientific validity of common orthopedic tests. *Arch Phys Med Rehabil.* 2003;84(4):592-603.

Quarles JD, Hosey RG. Medial and lateral collateral injuries: prognosis and treatment. *Prim Care.* 2004;31(4):957-975, ix.

KNEE

McMURRAY TEST

TEST POSITIONING

The subject lies supine. The examiner stands with the distal hand grasping the subject's heel or distal leg (medially), and the proximal hand on the subject's knee with the fingers palpating the medial and lateral joint lines (Figure K10-29A).

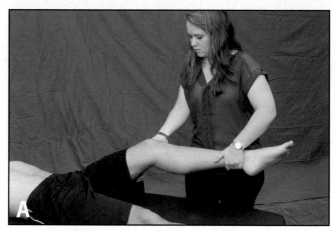

Figure K10-29A.

ACTION

With the knee as fully flexed as possible, externally rotate the tibia (Figure K10-29B), introduce a valgus force, and extend the knee (medial meniscus). Repeat with the tibia internally rotated and a varus force applied to the knee (lateral meniscus) (Figure K10-29C).

KNEE

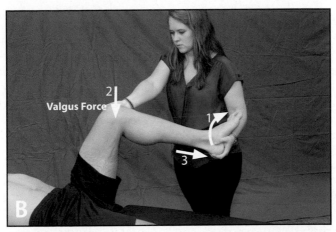

Figure K10-29B.

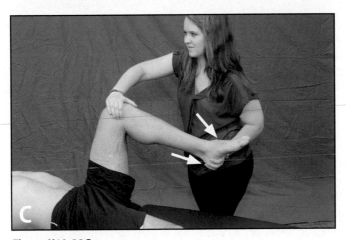

Figure K10-29C.

KNEE

POSITIVE FINDING

A "click" along the medial joint line is indicative of a medial meniscus tear. Likewise, a "click" along the lateral joint line is indicative of a lateral meniscus tear.

SPECIAL CONSIDERATIONS/COMMENTS

The examiner must not mistake a patellar "click" or "pop" for meniscal pathology. It may be difficult to accurately perform this test if there is a flap tear of the meniscus or excessive joint swelling that is limiting range of motion. The examiner should also be sensitive with palpation along the joint line because this can cause significant pain to the subject (especially if a meniscal tear is accompanied by a collateral ligament injury).

EVIDENCE

	Hing et al (2009)
Study design	Systematic review
Conditions evaluated	Meniscal pathology
Study number	9
Reliability	Not evaluated
Sensitivity	27 to 71
Specificity	29 to 96

REFERENCES

Akseki D, Pinar H, Karaoğlan O. The accuracy of the clinical diagnosis of meniscal tears with or without associated anterior cruciate ligament tears [article in Turkish]. *Acta Orthop Traumatol Turc.* 2003;37(3):193-198.

Evans PJ, Bell GD, Frank C. Prospective evaluation of the McMurray test. *Am J Sports Med.* 1993;21(4):604-608.

Fowler PJ, Lubliner JA. The predictive value of five clinical signs in the evaluation of meniscal pathology. *Arthroscopy.* 1989;5(3):184-186.

Hing W, White S, Reid D, Marshall R. Validity of the McMurray's Test and modified versions of the test: a systematic literature review. *J Man Manip Ther.* 2009;17(1):22-35.

Kim SJ, Min BH, Han DY. Paradoxical phenomena of the McMurray test. An arthroscopic investigation. *Am J Sports Med.* 1996;24(1):83-87.

Kurosaka M, Yagi M, Yoshiya S, Muratsu H, Mizuno K. Efficacy of the axially loaded pivot shift test for the diagnosis of a meniscal tear. *Int Orthop.* 1999;23(5):271-274.

McMurray TP. The semilunar cartilages. *Br J Surg.* 1942;29:407-414.

Metcalf MH, Barrett GR. Prospective evaluation of 1485 meniscal tear patterns in patients with stable knees. *Am J Sports Med.* 2004;32(3):675-680.

Nevsímal L, Skoták M, Míka P, Běhounek J. Clinical examination of menisci in the era of arthroscopy [article in Czech]. *Acta Chir Orthop Traumatol Cech.* 2002;69(2):88-94.

Pookarnjanamorakot C, Korsantirat T, Woratanarat P. Meniscal lesions in the anterior cruciate insufficient knee: the accuracy of clinical evaluation. *J Med Assoc Thai.* 2004;87(6):618-623.

Scholten RJ, Devillé WL, Opstelten W, Bijl D, van der Plas CG, Bouter LM. The accuracy of physical diagnostic tests for assessing meniscal lesions of the knee: a meta-analysis. *J Fam Pract.* 2001;50(11):938-944.

Stratford PW, Binkley J. A review of the McMurray test: definition, interpretation, and clinical usefulness. *J Orthop Sports Phys Ther.* 1995;22(3):116-120.

APLEY COMPRESSION TEST

TEST POSITIONING

The subject lies prone with the test knee flexed to 90 degrees. The examiner stands with the proximal hand on the subject's distal thigh for stabilization and the distal hand on the subject's heel (Figure K10-30A).

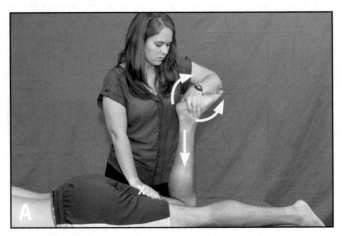

Figure K10-30A.

ACTION

With the distal hand, medially and laterally rotate the tibia while applying a downward force through the heel.

POSITIVE FINDING

Pain, clicking, and/or restriction is indicative of either a medial or lateral meniscus tear, depending on the location of symptoms.

KNEE

SPECIAL CONSIDERATIONS/COMMENTS

The test may be repeated with a distraction force (eg, Apley Distraction Test) applied to the ankle with the distal hand (Figure K10-30B). An increase and/or change in location of pain is more indicative of ligamentous versus meniscal pathology. Pain and/or clicking with a compression test that is followed by an absence of the same symptoms with a distraction test is most likely indicative of meniscal pathology.

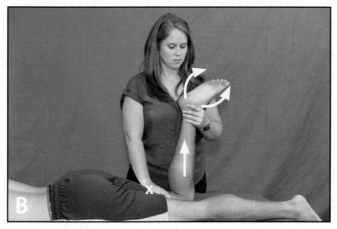

Figure K10-30B.

EVIDENCE

	Malanga et al (2003)	Pookarnjanamorakot et al (2004)
Study design	Systematic review	Cross-sectional
Conditions evaluated	Meniscal pathologies	Meniscal injuries
Study number	2	
Sample size		100
Reliability	Not evaluated	Not evaluated
Sensitivity	13 to 16	16
Specificity	80 to 90	100

REFERENCES

Fowler PJ, Lubliner JA. The predictive value of five clinical signs in the evaluation of meniscal pathology. *Arthroscopy.* 1989;5(3):184-186.

Kurosaka M, Yagi M, Yoshiya S, Muratsu H, Mizuno K. Ffficacy of the axially loaded pivot shift test for the diagnosis of a meniscal tear. *Int Orthop.* 1999;23(5):271-274.

Malanga GA, Andrus S, Nadler SF, McLean J. Physical examination of the knee: a review of the original test description and scientific validity of common orthopedic tests. *Arch Phys Med Rehabil.* 2003;84(4):592-603.

Pookarnjanamorakot C, Korsantirat T, Woratanarat P. Meniscal lesions in the anterior cruciate insufficient knee: the accuracy of clinical evaluation. *J Med Assoc Thai.* 2004;87(6):618-623.

STEINMAN'S TENDERNESS DISPLACEMENT TEST

TEST POSITIONING

The subject lies supine with the knee in full extension. The examiner places the proximal hand under the involved knee and grasps the ankle with the distal hand (Figure K10-31A).

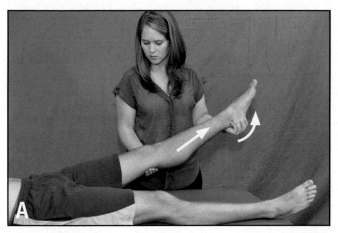

Figure K10-31A.

ACTION

The examiner passively moves the subject's involved knee into various ranges of knee flexion, followed by a dynamic movement into internal rotation (Figure K10-31B) and external rotation (Figure K10-31C).

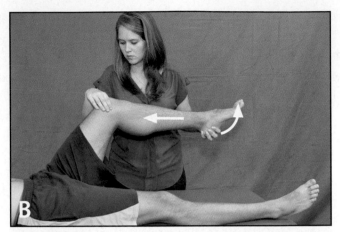

Figure K10-31B.

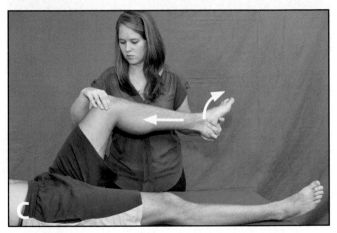

Figure K10-31C.

POSITIVE FINDING

A subject who either complains of pain during the rotational component or lacks full flexion may have a meniscal tear.

SPECIAL CONSIDERATIONS/COMMENTS

It is important to maintain quadriceps and hamstring muscle relaxation during this test. If the subject is unable to obtain full flexion, the examiner may want to perform passive internal and external rotation at the point of maximal available flexion and assess for any reproduction of pain.

EVIDENCE

	Pookarnjanamorakot et al (2004)
Study design	Cross-sectional
Conditions evaluated	Meniscal injuries
Sample size	100
Reliability	Not evaluated
Sensitivity	28 to 29
Specificity	100

REFERENCES

Dervin GF, Stiell IG, Rody K, Grabowski J. Effect of arthroscopic debridement for osteoarthritis of the knee on health-related quality of life. *J Bone Joint Surg Am.* 2003;85-A(1):10-19.

Pookarnjanamorakot C, Korsantirat T, Woratanarat P. Meniscal lesions in the anterior cruciate insufficient knee: the accuracy of clinical evaluation. *J Med Assoc Thai.* 2004;87(6):618-623.

Nevsímal L, Skoták M, Míka P, Běhounek J. Clinical examination of menisci in the era of arthroscopy [article in Czech]. *Acta Chir Orthop Traumatol Cech.* 2002;69(2):88-94.

KNEE

THESSALY TEST

TEST POSITIONING

The subject stands on one leg with the knee slightly flexed (5 degrees) (Figure K10-32A). The examiner holds both of the subject's hands to provide support and balance.

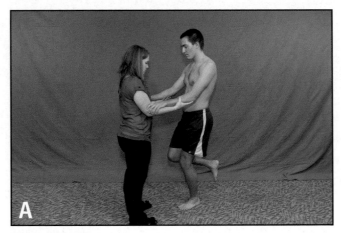

Figure K10-32A.

ACTION

The subject twists back and forth 3 times, rotating the knees and body internally and externally (Figures K10-32B through K10-32D).

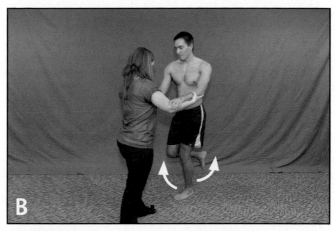

Figure K10-32B.

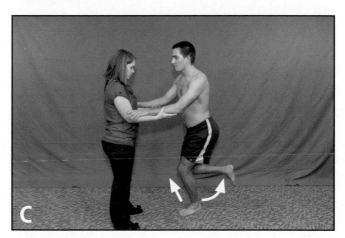

Figure K10-32C.

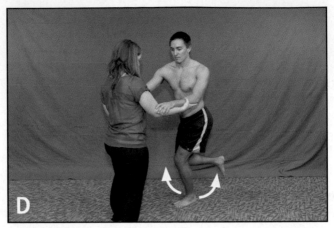

Figure K10-32D.

POSITIVE FINDING

Reports from the subject of medial or lateral joint line pain or the sensation of catching or locking suggests a positive test and an injury to a meniscus.

SPECIAL CONSIDERATIONS/COMMENTS

Once the test is completed in 5 degrees of flexion, it is repeated in 20 degrees of flexion. Additionally, it is important to start this test on the uninvolved leg first and then proceed to the involved leg.

Evidence

	Karachalios et al (2005)	Mirzatolooei et al (2010)	Snoeker et al (2015)
Study design	Diagnostic accuracy	Diagnostic accuracy	Reliability and diagnostic accuracy
Conditions evaluated	Meniscal tears	Meniscal tears	Meniscal tears
Sample size	213	80	121
Reliability	Not evaluated	Not evaluated	Kappa = .54
Sensitivity	5 degrees flexion = 65 20 degrees flexion = 80	20 degrees flexion = 79	20 degrees flexion = 67 and 51
Specificity	5 degrees flexion = 83 20 degrees flexion = 91	20 degrees flexion = 40	20 degrees flexion = 38 and 44

References

Karachalios T, Hantes M, Zibis AH, Zachos V, Karantanas AH, Malizos KN. Diagnostic accuracy of a new clinical test (the Thessaly test) for early detection of meniscal tears. *J Bone Joint Surg Am.* 2005;87(5):955-962.

Mirzatolooei F, Yekta Z, Bayazidchi M, Ershadi S, Afshar A. Validation of the Thessaly test for detecting meniscal tears in anterior cruciate deficient knees. *Knee.* 2010;17(3):221-223.

Snoeker BA, Lindeboom R, Zwinderman AH, Vincken PW, Jansen JA, Lucas C. Detecting meniscal tears in primary care: reproducibility and accuracy of 2 weight-bearing and 1 non-weight-bearing tests [published online ahead of print July 10, 2015]. *J Orthop Sports Phys Ther.* doi:10.2519/jospt.2015.5712.

KNEE

OBER'S TEST

TEST POSITIONING

The subject lies on the side with the hips and knees extended so the test leg is superior to the nontest leg. The examiner stands behind the subject with the proximal hand stabilizing the pelvis and the distal hand supporting the lower leg (Figure K10-33A). The knee of the test leg is flexed to 90 degrees.

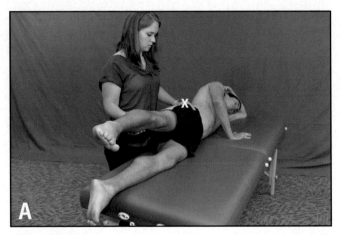

Figure K10-33A.

ACTION

The knee of the test leg is flexed to 90 degrees. With the pelvis stabilized to prevent rolling, abduct and extend the test hip to position the iliotibial band behind the greater trochanter (Figure K10-33B). Then allow the leg to slowly lower (adduct).

KNEE

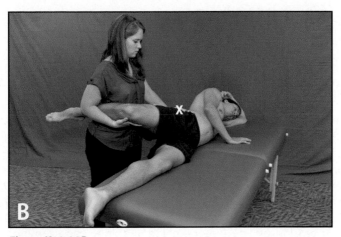

Figure K10-33B.

Positive Finding

The inability of the leg to adduct and touch the table is indicative of iliotibial band (particularly the tensor fasciae latae) tightness. The leg will react like a "springboard" because the leg remains abducted in mid-air (Figure K10-33C).

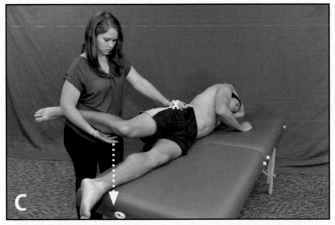

Figure K10-33C. Note: The weight of the leg drops the leg toward the table.

SPECIAL CONSIDERATIONS/COMMENTS

It is important to apply a downward force on the ilium near the crest while allowing the leg to adduct. This will prevent lateral tilting (ie, inferior movement) of the pelvis on the side of the test leg, which could give a false-negative result. Additionally, it is important to ensure complete relaxation of the hip abductor muscles. It may be helpful to have the subject actively adduct the test leg into the support hand and then relax to inhibit hip abductor muscle guarding. This test was originally described by Ober to be performed with the knee flexed to 90 degrees. However, it has been modified (ie, Modified Ober's Test) because it is believed that a greater stretch is placed on the iliotibial band when the knee is in an extended position. Furthermore, performing this test with the knee in flexion places greater tension on the femoral nerve, requiring the examiner to be cognizant of associated neurological complaints.

EVIDENCE

	Reese and Bandy (2003)	Ferber et al (2010)
Study design	Reliability	Cross-sectional
Conditions evaluated	Iliotibial band tightness	Iliotibial band tightness
Sample size	61	300
Reliability	Intrarater reliability = .90	Interrater agreement = 97.6%
Sensitivity	Not evaluated	Not evaluated
Specificity	Not evaluated	Not evaluated

REFERENCES

Ferber R, Kendall KD, McElroy L. Normative and critical criteria for iliotibial band and iliopsoas muscle flexibility. *J Athl Train*. 2010;45(4):344-348.

Fredericson M, White JJ, Macmahon JM, Andriachi TP. Quantitative analysis of the relative effectiveness of 3 iliotibial band stretches. *Arch Phys Med Rehabil*. 2002;83(5):589-592.

Gajdosik RL, Sandler MM, Marr HL. Influence of knee positions and gender on the Ober test for length of the iliotibial band. *Clin Biomech (Bristol, Avon).* 2003;18(1):77-79.

Gautam VK, Anand S. A new test for estimating iliotibial band contracture. *J Bone Joint Surg Br.* 1998;80(3):474-475.

Margo K, Drezner J, Motzkin D. Evaluation and management of hip pain: an algorithmic approach. *J Fam Pract.* 2003;52(8):607-617.

Melchione WE, Sullivan MS. Reliability of measurements obtained by use of an instrument designed to indirectly measure iliotibial band length. *J Orthop Sports Phys Ther.* 1993;18(3):511-515.

Ober FB. The role of the iliotibial and fascia lata as a factor in the causation of low-back disabilities and sciatica. *J Bone Joint Surg.* 1936;18:105.

Reese NB, Bandy WD. Use of an inclinometer to measure flexibility of the iliotibial band using the Ober test and the modified Ober test: differences in magnitude and reliability of measurements. *J Orthop Sports Phys Ther.* 2003;33(6):326-330.

Winslow J, Yoder E. Patellofemoral pain in female ballet dancers: correlation with iliotibial band tightness and tibial external rotation. *J Orthop Sports Phys Ther.* 1995;22(1):18-21.

QUAD ACTIVE TEST

TEST POSITIONING

The subject lies supine and flexes the knee to 90 degrees (Figure K10-34). The examiner stabilizes the subject's foot on the table.

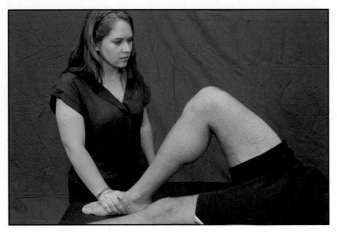

Figure K10-34.

ACTION

The examiner asks the subject to contract or "fire" the quadriceps while the examiner applies counter pressure on the ankle.

POSITIVE FINDING

A PCL tear is suggested when the tibia is displaced by more than 2 mm during the action of the test.

SPECIAL CONSIDERATIONS/COMMENTS

The examiner should closely watch the positioning of the subject's knee throughout the motion to accurately evaluate displacement of the tibia.

KNEE

EVIDENCE

	Malanga et al (2003)
Study design	Systematic review
Conditions evaluated	PCL injuries
Study number	2
Reliability	Not evaluated
Sensitivity	54 to 98
Specificity	97 to 100

REFERENCES

Malanga GA, Andrus S, Nadler SF, McLean J. Physical examination of the knee: a review of the original test description and scientific validity of common orthopedic tests. *Arch Phys Med Rehabil.* 2003;84(4):592-603.

Rubinstein RA Jr, Shelbourne KD, McCarroll JR, VanMeter CD, Rettig AC. The accuracy of the clinical examination in the setting of posterior cruciate ligament injuries. *Am J Sports Med.* 1994;22(4):550-557.

LELLI TEST FOR
ANTERIOR CRUCIATE LIGAMENT (ACL) INJURIES

TEST POSITIONING

The subject lies supine on an examination table with the legs extended. The examiner places a fist under the calf of the involved leg, ensuring that the subject's heel remains on the exam table.

ACTION

The examiner uses his or her other hand to place a downward, light force on the distal quadriceps of the involved leg (Figure K10-35).

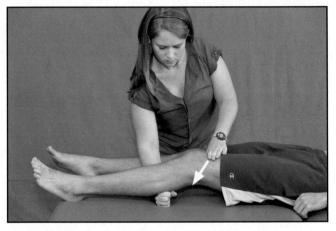

Figure K10-35.

POSITIVE FINDING

The Lelli Test is positive when the downward, light force on the quadriceps does not result in the heel lifting off the table. A positive test suggests a complete rupture of the ACL. If the foot lifts off the table, then the test suggests there is not a rupture of the ACL.

SPECIAL CONSIDERATIONS/COMMENTS

The fist under the calf serves as a fulcrum. Pay attention to the amount of force placed on the involved quadriceps. If there is no rupture, even a very small amount of force will result in the heel lifting off the table. If the ACL is ruptured, even a large force will not result in the heel lifting off the table. This test is also called the Lever Sign.

EVIDENCE

	Lelli et al (2014)
Study design	Diagnostic accuracy
Conditions evaluated	ACL tears
Sample size	400
Reliability	Not evaluated
Sensitivity	100
Specificity	100

REFERENCE

Lelli A, Di Turi RP, Spenciner DB, Dòmini M. The "Lever Sign": a new clinical test for the diagnosis of anterior cruciate ligament rupture [published online ahead of print December 25, 2014]. *Knee Surg Sports Traumatol Arthrosc.* DOI:10.1007/s00167-014-3490-7.

KNEE

Please see videos on the accompanying website at
www.healio.com/books/specialtestsvideos

Section

11

Ankle and Foot

Guide to Figures

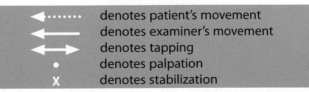

denotes patient's movement
denotes examiner's movement
denotes tapping
denotes palpation
denotes stabilization

Konin JG, Lebsack D, Snyder Valier AR, Isear JA Jr.
Special Tests for Orthopedic Examination, Fourth Edition (pp 363-391).
© 2016 SLACK Incorporated.

HOMANS' SIGN

TEST POSITIONING

The subject lies supine on a table.

ACTION

With the knee of the involved side fully extended, the examiner passively dorsiflexes the subject's foot (Figure AF11-1A).

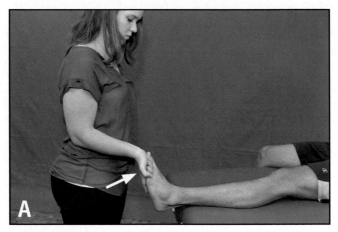

Figure AF11-1A.

POSITIVE FINDING

A production of pain in the calf that is brought on by the passive stretch of the foot into a dorsiflexed position is a positive sign for thrombophlebitis.

SPECIAL CONSIDERATIONS/COMMENTS

Pain may also be elicited on palpation of the calf in conjunction with the passive stretch (Figure AF11-1B). A positive finding indicates a life-threatening condition that should be addressed by appropriate medical personnel immediately.

ANKLE AND FOOT

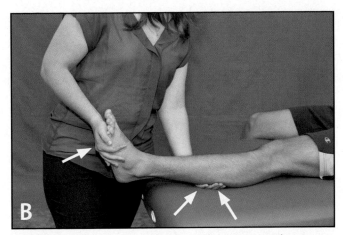

Figure AF11-1B. Note: The examiner applies pressure on the gastrocnemius muscle while passively moving the ankle into dorsiflexion.

REFERENCES

Cranley JJ, Canos AJ, Sull WJ. The diagnosis of deep venous thrombosis. Fallibility of clinical symptoms and signs. *Arch Surg.* 1976;111(1):34-36.

Henriet JP. Pain in venous thrombosis of the leg [article in French]. *Phlebologie.* 1992;45(1):67-76.

Levi M, Hart W, Büller HR. Physical examination—the significance of Homan's sign [article in Dutch]. *Ned Tijdschr Geneeskd.* 1999;143(37):1861-1863.

Matthewson M. A Homans' sign is an effective method of diagnosing thrombophlebitis in bedridden patients. *Crit Care Nurs.* 1983;3(4):64-65.

Ng KC. Deep vein thrombosis: a study in clinical diagnosis. *Singapore Med J.* 1994;35(3):286-289.

Sandler DA. Homan's sign and medical education. *Lancet.* 1985; 2(8464):1130-1131.

Wang CJ, Wang JW, Chen LM, et al. Deep vein thrombosis after total knee arthroplasty. *J Formos Med Assoc.* 2000;99(11):848-853.

ANTERIOR DRAWER TEST

TEST POSITIONING

The subject is seated at the end of a table with the knee flexed and the involved foot relaxed in slight plantar flexion. The examiner stabilizes the tibia and fibula with one hand and grasps the calcaneus with the other (Figure AF11-2A). This may also be performed with the subject in a prone position (Figure AF11-2B).

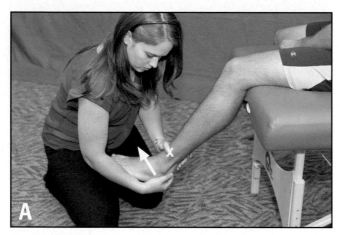

Figure AF11-2A.

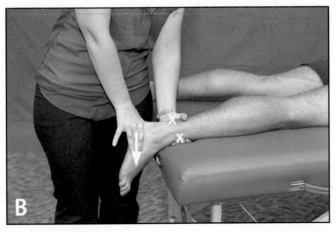

Figure AF11-2B.

ACTION

While ensuring stabilization of the distal tibia and fibula, the examiner applies an anterior force to the calcaneus and talus.

POSITIVE FINDING

Anterior translation of the talus away from the ankle mortise that is greater on the involved side, opposed to the noninvolved side, indicates a positive sign for a possible anterior talofibular ligament sprain.

SPECIAL CONSIDERATIONS/COMMENTS

The knee is flexed to 90 degrees to reduce the tension on the gastrocnemius muscle. This test should be performed bilaterally for comparison. Swelling within the ankle joint may reduce the ability to translate the talus anteriorly. A modified version can be performed in the prone position.

ANKLE AND FOOT

EVIDENCE

	Schwieterman et al (2013)	Sman et al (2013)
Study design	Systematic review	Systematic review
Conditions evaluated	Ankle/lower leg pathologies	Ankle syndesmosis injury
Study number	1	1
Sample size	20	21
Reliability	Not evaluated	Intrarater reliability: 46% to 92% agreement Interrater reliability: ICC = .06
Sensitivity	51	36
Specificity	100	43

REFERENCES

Bahr R, Peña F, Shine J, et al. Mechanics of the anterior drawer and talar tilt tests. A cadaveric study of lateral ligament injuries of the ankle. *Acta Orthop Scand.* 1997;68(5):435-441.

Beumer A, van Hemert WL, Swierstra BA, Jasper LE, Belkoff SM. A biomechanical evaluation of clinical stress tests for syndesmotic ankle instability. *Foot Ankle Int.* 2003;24(4):358-363.

Corazza F, O'Connor JJ, Leardini A, Parenti Castelli V. Ligament fibre recruitment and forces for the anterior drawer test at the human ankle joint. *J Biomech.* 2003;36(3):363-372.

Fujii T, Luo ZP, Kitaoka HB, An KN. The manual stress test may not be sufficient to differentiate ankle ligament injuries. *Clin Biomech (Bristol, Avon).* 2000;15(8):619-623.

Hertel J, Denegar CR, Monroe M, Stokes WL. Talocrucral and subtalar joint instability after lateral ankle sprain. *Med Sci Sports Exerc.* 1999;31(11):1501-1508.

Kanbe K, Hasegawa A, Nakajima Y, Takagishi K. The relationship of the anterior drawer sign to the shape of the tibial plafond in chronic lateral instability of the ankle. *Foot Ankle Int.* 2002;23(2):118-122.

Kerkhoffs GM, Blankevoort L, Schreurs AW, Jaspers JE, van Dijk CN. An instrumented, dynamic test for anterior laxity of the ankle joint complex. *J Biomech.* 2002;35(12):1665-1670.

Liu W, Maitland ME, Nigg BM. The effect of axial load on the in vivo anterior drawer test of the ankle joint complex. *Foot Ankle Int.* 2000;21(5):420-426.

Lynch SA. Assessment of the injured ankle in the athlete. *J Athl Train.* 2002;37(4):406-412.

Ray RG, Christensen JC, Gusman DN. Critical evaluation of anterior drawer measurement methods in the ankle. *Clin Orthop Relat Res.* 1997;(334):215-224.

Schwieterman B, Haas D, Columber K, Knupp D, Cook C. Diagnostic accuracy of physical examination tests of the ankle/foot complex: a systematic review. *Int J Sports Phys Ther.* 2013;8(4):416-426.

Sman AD, Hiller CE, Refshauge KM. Diagnostic accuracy of clinical tests for diagnosis of ankle syndesmosis injury: a systematic review. *Br J Sports Med.* 2013;47(10):620-628.

Stiell IG, McKnight RD, Greenberg GH, Nair RC, McDowell I, Wallace GJ. Interobserver agreement in the examination of acute ankle injury patients. *Am J Emerg Med.* 1992;10(1):14-17.

Tohyama H, Beynnon BD, Renström PA, Theis MJ, Fleming BC, Pope MH. Biomechanical analysis of the ankle anterior drawer test for anterior talofibular ligament injuries. *J Orthop Res.* 1995;13(4):609-614.

Tohyama H, Yasuda K, Ohkoshi Y, Beynnon BD, Renström PA. Anterior drawer test for acute anterior talofibular ligament injuries of the ankle. How much load should be applied during the test? *Am J Sports Med* 2003;31(2):226-232.

TALAR TILT TEST (INVERSION)

TEST POSITIONING

The subject lies on the uninvolved side on a table with the involved foot relaxed and the knee slightly flexed. The examiner stabilizes the distal tibia with one hand while grasping the talus with the other.

ACTION

The examiner first places the foot in the anatomical position (neutral plantar flexion and dorsiflexion). The examiner then tilts the talus into an adducted position (Figure AF11-3).

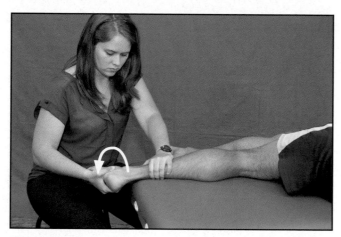

Figure AF11-3.

POSITIVE FINDING

Range of motion in the adducted position on the involved foot greater than that of the noninvolved foot reveals a positive test. This may be indicative of a tear of the calcaneofibular ligament of the ankle.

SPECIAL CONSIDERATIONS/COMMENTS

The knee is flexed to 90 degrees to reduce the tension on the gastrocnemius muscle. This test should be performed bilaterally for comparison. Performing this test with the ankle in a more plantar flexed position places less stress on the calcaneofibular ligament and instead may stress the anterior talofibular ligament. Swelling within the ankle joint may reduce the ability to translate the talus.

EVIDENCE

	Schwieterman et al (2013)
Study design	Systematic review
Conditions evaluated	Ankle/lower leg pathologies
Study number	1
Sample size	20
Reliability	Not evaluated
Sensitivity	50
Specificity	88

REFERENCES

Bahr R, Peña F, Shine J, et al. Mechanics of the anterior drawer and talar tilt tests. A cadaveric study of lateral ligament injuries of the ankle. *Acta Orthop Scand.* 1997;68(5):435-441.

Fujii T, Luo ZP, Kitaoka HB, An KN. The manual stress test may not be sufficient to differentiate ankle ligament injuries. *Clin Biomech (Bristol, Avon).* 2000;15(8):619-623.

Gaebler C, Kukla C, Breitenseher MJ, et al. Diagnosis of lateral ankle ligament injuries: comparison between talar tilt, MRI, and operative findings in 112 athletes. *Acta Orthop Scand.* 1997;68(3):286-290.

Glasgow M, Jackson A, Jamieson A. Instability of the ankle after injury to the lateral ligament. *J Bone Joint Br.* 1980;62(2):196-200.

Hertel J, Denegar CR, Monroe MM, Stokes WL. Talocrucral and subtalar joint instability after lateral ankle sprain. *Med Sci Sports Exerc.* 1999;31(11):1501-1508.

Hollis JM, Blasier RD, Flahiff CM. Simulated lateral ankle ligamentous injury. Change in ankle stability. *Am J Sports Med.* 1995;23(6):672-677.

Schwieterman B, Haas D, Columber K, Knupp D, Cook C. Diagnostic accuracy of physical examination tests of the ankle/foot complex: a systematic review. *Int J Sports Phys Ther.* 2013;8(4):416-426.

TALAR TILT TEST (EVERSION)

TEST POSITIONING

The subject lies on the involved side on a table with the involved foot relaxed and the knee slightly flexed. The examiner stabilizes the distal tibia with one hand while grasping the talus with the other.

ACTION

The examiner first places the foot in the anatomical position (neutral plantar flexion and dorsiflexion). The examiner then tilts the talus into an abducted position (Figure AF11-4).

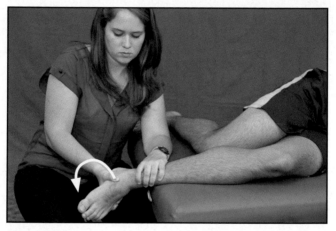

Figure AF11-4.

POSITIVE FINDING

Range of motion in the abducted position on the involved foot greater than that of the noninvolved foot reveals a positive test. This may be indicative of a tear of the deltoid ligament of the ankle.

Special Considerations/Comments

The knee is flexed to 90 degrees to reduce the tension on the gastrocnemius muscle. This test should be performed bilaterally for comparison. Performing this test with the ankle in varying degrees of plantar flexion may assess different components of the deltoid ligament. Swelling within the ankle joint may reduce the ability to translate the talus.

References

Fujii T, Luo ZP, Kitaoka HB, An KN. The manual stress test may not be sufficient to differentiate ankle ligament injuries. *Clin Biomech (Bristol, Avon)*. 2000;15(8):619-623.

Leith JM, McConkey JP, Li D, Masri B. Valgus stress radiography in normal ankles. *Foot Ankle Int.* 1997;18(10):654-657.

THOMPSON TEST

TEST POSITIONING

The subject lies prone on a table with the heels placed over the edge of the table.

ACTION

With the gastrocnemius-soleus complex relaxed, the examiner squeezes the belly of these muscles (Figure AF11-5).

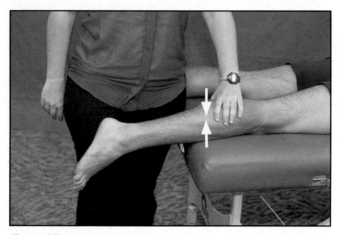

Figure AF11-5.

POSITIVE FINDING

When squeezing the calf muscles, a normal response would be to have the foot plantar flex. Therefore, an absence of plantar flexion on squeezing would be a positive test, indicating a possible rupture of the Achilles tendon.

ANKLE
AND FOOT

EVIDENCE

	Schwieterman et al (2013)
Study design	Systematic review
Conditions evaluated	Ankle/lower leg pathologies
Study number	1
Sample size	161
Reliability	Not evaluated
Sensitivity	96
Specificity	93

REFERENCES

O'Brien T. The needle test for complete rupture of the Achilles' tendon. *J Bone Joint Surg Am.* 1984;66(7):1099-1101.

Schwieterman B, Haas D, Columber K, Knupp D, Cook C. Diagnostic accuracy of physical examination tests of the ankle/foot complex: a systematic review. *Int J Sports Phys Ther.* 2013;8(4):416-426.

Thompson TC. A test for rupture of the tendo achillis. *Acta Orthop Scand.* 1962;32:461-465.

Thompson TC, Doherty JH. Spontaneous rupture of tendon of the Achilles: a new clinical diagnostic test. *J Trauma.* 1962;2:126-129.

ANKLE
AND FOOT

TAP OR PERCUSSION TEST

TEST POSITIONING

The subject lies supine with the affected leg extended and the ankle/foot just off the examining table. The examiner stands at the end of the table next to the subject's foot.

ACTION

The examiner positions the subject's ankle into a maximal dorsiflexion to optimize joint congruency and applies a firm tap to the bottom of the subject's heel (Figure AF11-6).

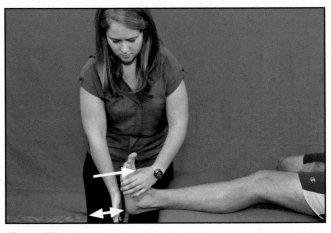

Figure AF11-6.

POSITIVE FINDING

Pain at the site of injury is indicative of a fracture. The vibration of tapping along the long axis of the bones will exaggerate pain at the fracture site.

SPECIAL CONSIDERATIONS/COMMENTS

This test should not be performed if there is an obvious deformity.

FEISS LINE

TEST POSITIONING

The subject sits on the examining table with the involved leg extended. The examiner places a mark at the tip of the medial malleolus and at the base of the first metatarsophalangeal joint. A line is then drawn between the 2 points and the examiner notes the position of the navicular tuberosity (Figure AF11-7A).

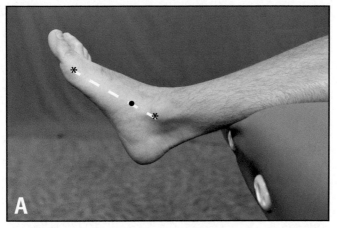

Figure AF11-7A. Note: The black circle denotes the location of the navicular bone.

ACTION

The subject is asked to stand with the feet 3 to 6 inches apart. The examiner ensures the marks are still positioned over the medial malleolus and first metatarsophalangeal joint and then again notes the position of the navicular tuberosity (Figure AF11-7B).

ANKLE AND FOOT

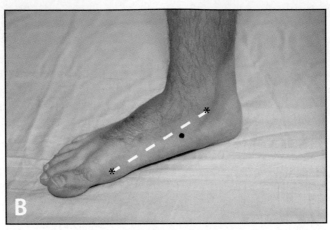

Figure AF11-7B. Note: The black circle denotes the location of the navicular bone.

POSITIVE FINDING

The navicular tuberosity should be in line with the other 2 points. If the navicular tuberosity is below the line while the subject is seated, the subject has congenital pes planus. If the navicular tuberosity is in line with the other 2 points while the subject is seated and it then falls below the line when the subject stands, functional pes planus is indicated.

SPECIAL CONSIDERATIONS/COMMENTS

This test may denote varying degrees of pes planus depending on how far the navicular drops to the floor. Pes planus may also be indicative of hyperpronation. A modified Feiss Line may be used in which the original positioning on the medial malleolus is moved to a parallel point on the Achilles tendon. The point on the base of the first metatarsophalangeal joint remains the same. The new Feiss Line goes through the navicular in the neutral foot. It is thought that this modification may make it easier for clinicians to identify high-arched (Feiss Line above the navicular) and low-arched (Feiss Line below the navicular) individuals.

EVIDENCE

	Spörndly-Nees et al (2011)
Study design	Reliability
Conditions evaluated	Navicular bone positioning
Sample size	43
Reliability	Intrarater reliability: ICC = .94
	Interrater reliability: ICC = .91
Sensitivity	Not evaluated
Specificity	Not evaluated

REFERENCES

Cashmere TB, Smith RM, Hunt AM. Medial longitudinal arch of the foot: stationary versus walking measures. *Foot Ankle Int.* 1999;20(2):112-118.

Gilmour JC, Burns Y. The measurement of the medial longitudinal arch in children. *Foot Ankle Int.* 2001;22(6):493-498.

Holmes C, Wilcox D, Fletcher J. Effect of a modified, low-dye medial longitudinal arch taping procedure on the subtler joint neutral position before and after light exercise. *J Orthop Sports Phys Ther.* 2002;32(5):194-201.

Komeda T, Tanaka Y, Takakura Y, Fujii T, Samoto N, Tamai S. Evaluation of the longitudinal arch of the foot with hallux valgus using a newly developed two-dimensional coordinate system. *J Orthop Sci.* 2001;6(2):110-118.

Spörndly-Nees S, Dåsberg B, Nielsen RO, Boesen MI, Langberg H. The navicular position test—a reliable measure of the navicular bone position during rest and loading. *Int J Sports Phys Ther.* 2011;6(3):199-205.

Williams D, McClay I. Measurements used to characterize the foot and the medial longitudinal arch: reliability and validity. *Phys Ther.* 2000;80(9):864-871.

Yakut Y, Otman S, Livanelioglu A, Uygur F. Evaluation of the foot arches in ballet dancers. *J Dance Med Sci.* 1997;1(4):139-142.

INTERDIGITAL NEUROMA TEST

TEST POSITIONING

The subject sits on the examining table with the involved leg extended. The examiner stands next to the involved foot and places one hand around the metatarsal heads (Figure AF11-8).

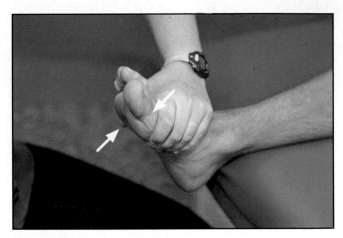

Figure AF11-8.

ACTION

The examiner squeezes the subject's metatarsal heads together and holds for 1 to 2 minutes.

POSITIVE FINDING

Pain, tingling, or numbness in the foot, toes, or ankle is indicative of an interdigital neuroma. If positive, the pain is usually relieved when pressure is released.

SPECIAL CONSIDERATIONS/COMMENTS

Pain between metatarsal heads is indicative of Morton's neuroma. The most common location is between the third and fourth metatarsal heads.

REFERENCES

Coughlin MJ, Pinsonneault T. Operative treatment of interdigital neuroma. A long-term follow-up study. *J Bone Joint Surg Am.* 2001;83(9):1321-1328.

Giannini S, Bacchini P, Ceccarelli F, Vannini F. Interdigital neuroma: clinical examination and histopathologic results in 63 cases treated with excision. *Foot Ankle Int.* 2004;25(2):79-84.

Stamatis ED, Karabalis C. Interdigital neuromas: current state of the art—surgical. *Foot Ankle Clin.* 2004;9(2):287-296.

Wu K. Morton neuroma and metatarsalgia. *Curr Opin Rheumatol.* 2000;12(2):131-142.

COMPRESSION (SQUEEZE) TEST

TEST POSITIONING

The subject lies supine with the affected leg extended and the ankle/foot just off the examining table. The examiner stands next to the subject's leg and notes where the pain originates.

ACTION

The examiner squeezes the tibia and fibula together at some point away from the painful area (Figure AF11-9).

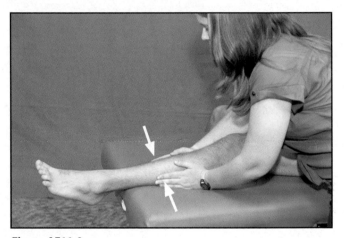

Figure AF11-9.

POSITIVE FINDING

Pain at the site of injury may be indicative of a fracture. Compression of the 2 bones may exaggerate pain at the fracture site.

SPECIAL CONSIDERATIONS/COMMENTS

This test should not be performed if there is an obvious deformity. A positive test is not exclusive of a fracture. It is recommended that an x-ray be obtained when suspicion of a fracture exists. A variation of the Compression Test, also called the Squeeze Test, can also be used to evaluate syndesmosis injuries. This modification requires that the compression be applied above the midpoint of the calf. A positive test with this modification is pain located over the syndesmosis ligaments.

EVIDENCE

	Schwieterman et al (2013)	Sman et al (2013)
Study design	Systematic review	Systematic review
Conditions evaluated	Ankle/lower leg pathologies	Syndesmosis injuries
Study number	1	2
Sample size	56	
Reliability	Not evaluated	Intrarater reliability: 88% to 92% agreement Interrater reliability: ICC = .46 to .49
Sensitivity	30	57 to 100
Specificity	93	14 to 63

REFERENCES

Schwieterman B, Haas D, Columber K, Knupp D, Cook C. Diagnostic accuracy of physical examination tests of the ankle/foot complex: a systematic review. *Int J Sports Phys Ther.* 2013;8(4):416-426.

Sman AD, Hiller CE, Refshauge KM. Diagnostic accuracy of clinical tests for diagnosis of ankle syndesmosis injury: a systematic review. *Br J Sports Med.* 2013;47(10):620-628.

LONG BONE COMPRESSION TEST

TEST POSITIONING

The subject sits with the affected leg extended and the foot off the end of the examining table. The examiner stands at the end of the table near the subject's foot.

ACTION

The examiner applies compression along the long axis of the bone of the toe or metatarsal being tested (Figure AF11-10).

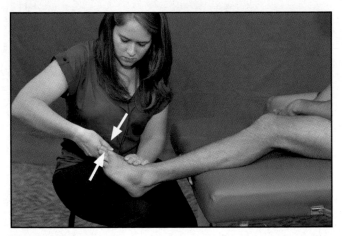

Figure AF11-10.

POSITIVE FINDING

Pain at the site of injury is indicative of a fracture.

SPECIAL CONSIDERATIONS/COMMENTS

This test should not be performed if there is an obvious deformity.

SWING TEST

TEST POSITIONING

The subject should sit with the foot over the edge of the table. The examiner stands in front of the subject and places both hands over the dorsum of the subject's foot to keep it parallel to the floor. The examiner palpates the anterior aspect of the subject's talus with the thumbs (Figure AF11-11A).

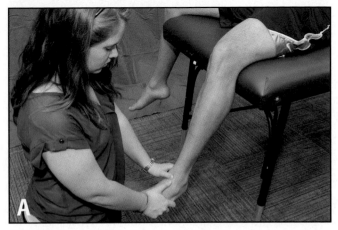

Figure AF11-11A.

ACTION

Passively plantar flex and dorsiflex the ankle and observe the level of movement, especially with dorsiflexion (Figure AF11-11B).

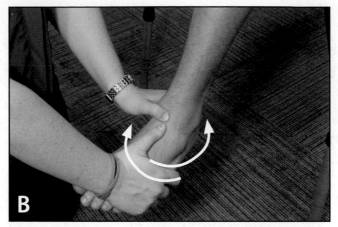

Figure AF11-11B.

POSITIVE FINDING

A positive test is revealed on resistance into dorsiflexion. This indicates posterior tibiotalar subluxation.

SPECIAL CONSIDERATIONS/COMMENTS

Imaging tests should always be considered when excessive joint motion is observed to be sure there is no underlying fracture.

KLEIGER'S TEST

TEST POSITIONING

The subject sits with the leg off of the table and the knee at 90 degrees of flexion. The examiner stabilizes the distal tibia and fibula with one hand and the medial and inferior aspects of the calcaneus with the other hand. The ankle should be in a neutrally aligned position (Figure AF11-12A).

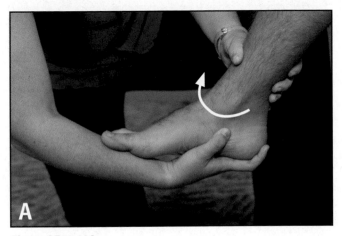

Figure AF11-12A.

ACTION

The examiner applies an externally rotated force on the calcaneus. The test is repeated with the ankle in a dorsiflexed position (Figure AF11-12B).

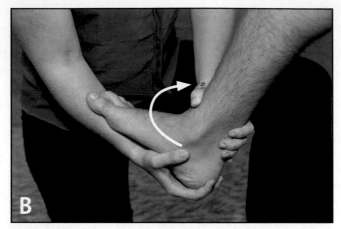

Figure AF11-12B.

POSITIVE FINDING

Complaints of pain along the medial aspect of the ankle when an externally rotated force is applied in neutral dorsiflexion may indicate a deltoid ligament injury. When the ankle is dorsiflexed and an externally rotated force is applied, pain may be present medially and slightly more proximally, indicating distal tibiofibular syndesmotic involvement.

SPECIAL CONSIDERATIONS/COMMENTS

The syndesmosis may be injured when the foot is fixated and a significant rotational force is applied. This is often referred to as a "high ankle sprain" and may be very painful to the subject when reproduction of the rotational torque is applied.

ANKLE AND FOOT

REFERENCES

Beumer A, van Hemert WL, Swierstra BA, Jasper LE, Belkoff SM. A biomechanical evaluation of clinical stress tests for syndesmotic ankle instability. *Foot Ankle Int.* 2003;24(4):358-363.

Candal-Couto JJ, Burrow D, Bromage S, Briggs PJ. Instability of the tibiofibular syndesmosis: have we been pulling in the wrong direction? *Injury.* 2004;35(8):814-818.

Kinoshita M, Okuda R, Morikawa J, Jotoku T, Abe M. The dorsiflexion-eversion test for diagnosis of tarsal tunnel syndrome. *J Bone Joint Surg.* 2001;83-A(12):1835-1839.

Seiler H. The upper ankle joint. Biomechanics and functional anatomy [article in German]. *Orthopade.* 1999;28(6):460-468.

TINEL'S SIGN

TEST POSITIONING

The subject typically lies supine.

ACTION

The examiner uses his or her finger to tap over the medial aspect of the ankle where the posterior tibial nerve is most superficial (Figure AF11-13).

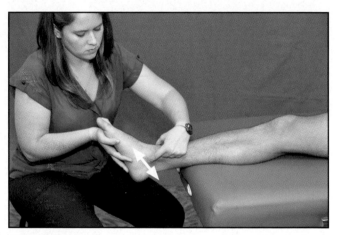

Figure AF11-13.

POSITIVE FINDING

Pain or tingling that radiates along the pathway of the posterior tibial nerve is indicative of potential tarsal tunnel syndrome. Compression of the posterior tibial nerve in the tarsal tunnel will result in referred symptoms to the medial and plantar regions of the foot.

ANKLE AND FOOT

SPECIAL CONSIDERATIONS/COMMENTS

A positive test simply refers to the fact that the posterior tibial nerve has been compromised. The nerve itself could be undergoing compression, as would be seen with inflammation within the tarsal tunnel, or it could be undergoing traction, as is the case with a hyper-pronated foot.

EVIDENCE

	Schwieterman et al (2013)
Study design	Systematic review
Conditions evaluated	Ankle/lower leg pathologies
Study number	1
Sample size	19
Reliability	Not evaluated
Sensitivity	58
Specificity	Not evaluated

REFERENCES

Bailie DS, Kelikian AS. Tarsal tunnel syndrome: diagnosis, surgical technique, and functional outcome. *Foot Ankle Int.* 1998;19(2):65-72.

Coughlin MJ, Pinsonneault T. Operative treatment of interdigital neuroma: a long-term follow-up study. *J Bone Joint Surg.* 2001;83-A(9):1321-1328.

Fabre T, Piton C, André D, Lasseur E, Durandeau A. Peroneal nerve entrapment. *J Bone Joint Surg Am.* 1998;80(1):47-53.

Schwieterman B, Haas D, Columber K, Knupp D, Cook C. Diagnostic accuracy of physical examination tests of the ankle/foot complex: a systematic review. *Int J Sports Phys Ther.* 2013;8(4):416-426.

Shookster L, Falke GI, Ducic I, Maloney CT Jr, Dellon AL. Fibromyalgia and Tinel's sign in the foot. *J Am Podiatr Med Assoc.* 2004;94(4):400-403.

ANKLE AND FOOT

Please see videos on the accompanying website at
www.healio.com/books/specialtestsvideos

Section
12

Contemporary
Special Tests

Guide to Figures

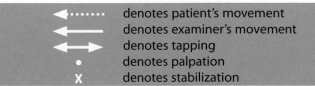

denotes patient's movement
denotes examiner's movement
denotes tapping
• denotes palpation
X denotes stabilization

Konin JG, Lebsack D, Snyder Valier AR, Isear JA Jr.
Special Tests for Orthopedic Examination, Fourth Edition (pp 393-406).
© 2016 SLACK Incorporated.

IMPINGEMENT REDUCTION TEST

TEST POSITIONING

The subject is seated or standing with the arm at rest and the shoulder internally rotated (Figure CST12-1A).

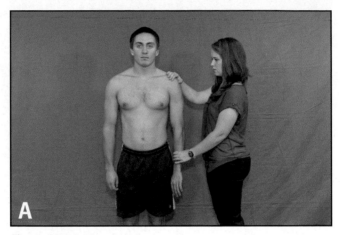

Figure CST12-1A.

ACTION

The examiner passively forward-flexes the involved arm while maintaining shoulder internal rotation (Figure CST12-1B). This motion is then repeated while the examiner applies an inferior glide to the humeral head (Figure CST12-1C).

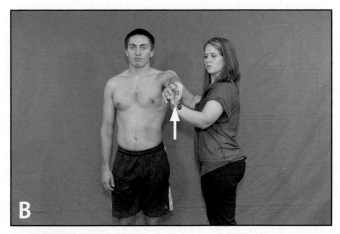

Figure CST12-1B.

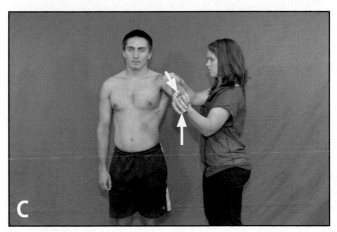

Figure CST12-1C.

Positive Finding

The reporting of shoulder joint pain is indicative of a positive test. Pain reported during passive shoulder flexion is indicative of a possible subacromial impingement. Absence of such pain on repeated passive flexion, accompanied by an inferior glide to the humeral head, confirms structural impingement. Pain reported with both passive shoulder flexion and passive shoulder flexion with an inferior humeral head glide reduces the likelihood of subacromial impingement and warrants further evaluative testing.

Special Considerations/Comments

This test can be modified either by testing in the frontal plane or the plane of the scapula or by placing the shoulder in external rotation to assess various components of the glenohumeral complex for impingement.

WALKING ARM STRESS (WAS) TEST

TEST POSITIONING

The subject lies relaxed and supine on the examination table with arms at side (Figure CST12-2A).

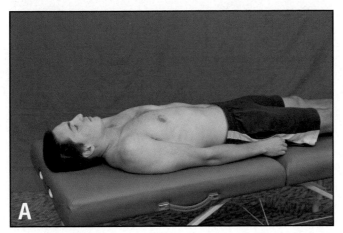

Figure CST12-2A.

ACTION

The examiner stands at the head of the examination table and places the palm of each hand under each of the subject's scapulae (Figure CST12-2B). The subject is asked to extend one arm into the table forcefully while the examiner simultaneously assesses the amount of pressure felt under the scapulae. The test is repeated with the other arm. The subject is asked to alternate extending each arm into the table while the examiner compares bilateral pressure applied to the palm of the hand.

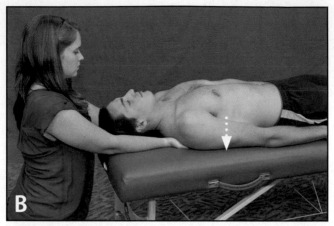

Figure CST12-2B.

POSITIVE FINDING

Lack of scapula pressure felt on the contralateral testing side is indicative of a decreased effort.

SPECIAL CONSIDERATIONS/COMMENTS

Subjects who apply forceful shoulder extension into the table will likely use the contralateral scapula for stabilization. This will be noted by the examiner. On the contrary, subjects who do not apply a true effort will tend to stabilize the central portion of the upper trunk, not applying unilateral pressure under the contralaterally tested scapula. This test should be used to consider malingering and not to rule out any specific pathology.

FINGER EXTENSION TEST

TEST POSITIONING

The subject is seated with the hand in a resting position.

ACTION

The examiner first attempts to passively extend the involved distal interphalangeal (DIP) or proximal interphalangeal (PIP) joint into full extension (Figure CST12-3A). The examiner then asks the subject to gently attempt to actively extend the involved DIP or PIP joint against minimal resistance provided by the examiner (Figure CST12-3B).

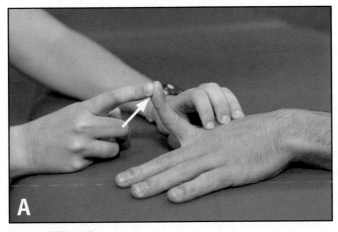

Figure CST12-3A.

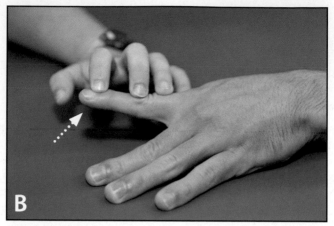

Figure CST12-3B.

Positive Finding

Inability to actively or passively extend the involved DIP or PIP joint is considered a positive test (Figure CST12-3C). If the joint is unable to be extended both actively and passively, one must consider capsuloligamentous restrictions or acute swelling and/or pain. The ability to extend the involved joint passively but inability to extend the same involved joint actively is likely indicative of an extensor tendon disruption.

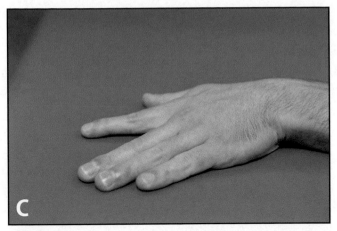

Figure CST12-3C.

Special Considerations/Comments

The examiner should apply only light resistance against active joint extension for the purposes of assessing any noticeable contraction. Moderate to maximal resistance is not encouraged because any tendon disruption may become complicated with increased contractile efforts. If a tendon disruption is suspected, this test should not be repeated for demonstration, confirmation, or educational purposes beyond what is necessary for clinical diagnosis.

FLEXOR PRONATOR SYNDROME TEST

TEST POSITIONING

The subject is seated with the involved forearm resting on a table with the elbow in a position of 90 degrees of flexion (Figure CST12-4A).

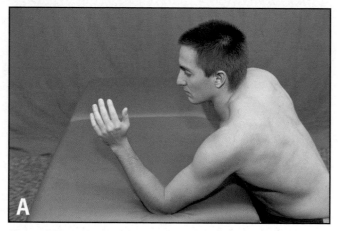

Figure CST12-4A.

ACTION

The examiner attempts to "shake hands" with the subject. The subject is then asked to pronate the forearm (Figure CST12-4B).

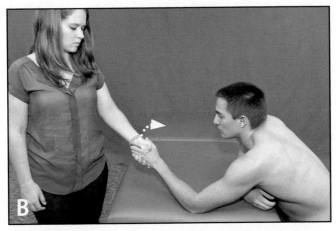

Figure CST12-4B.

POSITIVE FINDING

Pain and/or muscle weakness is considered a positive sign for a flexor pronator musculotendinous injury.

SPECIAL CONSIDERATIONS/COMMENTS

The examiner does not need to apply much resistance while the subject attempts to pronate the forearm. An acute inflammatory response will elicit a painful effort on the part of the subject.

TARSAL TWIST TEST

TEST POSITIONING

The patient is seated on a table with knees flexed to 90 degrees. The involved ankle is placed in neutral dorsiflexion/plantar flexion. The examiner stabilizes the rearfoot (subtalar joint) with one hand and grasps the forefoot with the opposite hand (Figure CST12-5A). The distal hand placement should be in the region of the tarsometatarsal joints.

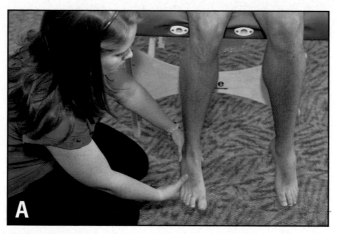

Figure CST12-5A.

ACTION

While ensuring stabilization of the subtalar joint, the examiner applies a medial rotatory force (Figure CST12-5B) and a lateral rotatory force (Figure CST12-5C) through the midfoot. The test is performed to stress the ligamentous stabilizers of the talocalcaneonavicular joint, the cuneonavicular joint, the calcaneocuboid joint, the cuboideonavicular joint, the cuneocuboid joint, the intercuneiform joint, and the tarsometatarsal joints.

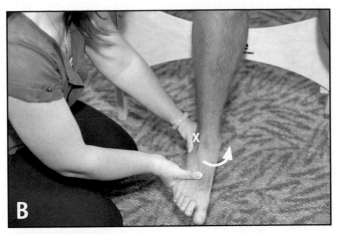

Figure CST12-5B.

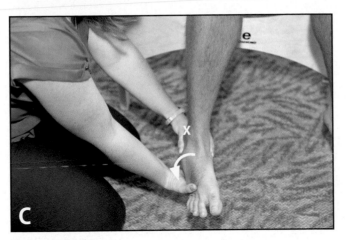

Figure CST12-5C.

POSITIVE FINDING

Pain in the region of the midfoot is a positive finding for a midfoot sprain. The location of the pain may assist the clinician in identifying the exact location of the injury with regard to the joints of the midfoot.

SPECIAL CONSIDERATIONS/COMMENTS

This test may also be performed with the patient in the supine or long-sitting position. This test should not be performed if there is obvious deformity present. Midfoot injuries are commonly found in association with lateral ankle sprains. This is particularly true when the ankle is in a plantar-flexed position and the midfoot is forced into a supination (twisting) motion. Additionally, injuries to the midfoot can result from repeated trauma, as seen in distance runners. Overuse injuries to the midfoot are most commonly associated with excessive pronation during gait.

Please see videos on the accompanying website at
www.healio.com/books/specialtestsvideos

CONTEMPORARY
SPECIAL TESTS

FINANCIAL DISCLOSURES

Jerome A. "Jai" Isear, Jr. has not disclosed any relevant financial relationships.

Dr. Jeff G. Konin has no financial or proprietary interest in the materials presented herein.

Dr. Denise Lebsack has no financial or proprietary interest in the materials presented herein.

Dr. Edward G. McFarland has no financial or proprietary interest in the materials presented herein.

Dr. Alison R. Snyder Valier has no financial or proprietary interest in the materials presented herein.

INDEX